Advanced Concepts of Personal Training
Lab Manual

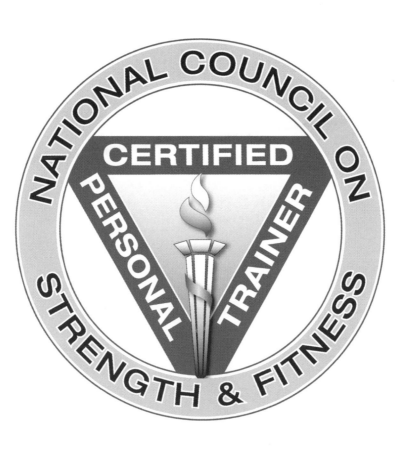

Brian D. Biagioli, EdD
Florida International University

Editorial Staff
Matthew Biagioli, MD
Wesley Smith, PhD
Sean Grieve, MS
Anthony Wyrwas, DC
Steven Wermus, MS

Book Development Staff
Paul Garbarino, MS
Tyler Poynton
B Glass Typography

Printed in the United States of America

Library of Congress Control Number: 2007926718

ISBN 978-0-9791696-2-5

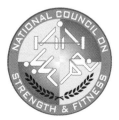

Table of Contents

Lab One
Functional Movement Application

Lab one corresponds to the following textbook readings:

Functional Anatomy	Chapter 1
Biomechanics	Chapter 2
Muscle Physiology	Chapter 3

Lab Description

All personal trainers must possess a thorough understanding of human anatomy to properly prescribe exercise. The human body is composed of a series of mechanical systems that work synergistically with one another to produce locomotion or movement. Understanding how these systems work will better allow the personal trainer to elicit the desired responses from his or her respective clientele.

The human body contains approximately 206 bones and over 700 different muscles. Lab one will provide you with an overview of the gross anatomical structures pertinent to human locomotion, activity, and exercise. Once proper anatomical identification can be made, movement terminology and the planes of motion will be reviewed and then applied through the performance of designated activities.

Explored Procedures

- Anatomical review and structure identification
- Analysis of exercise performance and appropriate use of movement terminology
- Identification of joint action and planes of movement used during exercise
- Review of stability requirements for select exercises

Lab Objectives

- Identify human skeletal and muscular structures
- Understand the application of anatomical movement terminology
- Be able to identify the muscle action, planes of movement, and prime mover activity during exercise
- Be able to identify the pelvic positions used during activity performance
- Identify factors that affect stability in human movement

Activity 1.1 Skeletal and Muscular Structure Identification

Activity Description

A step in understanding human movement and how it relates to exercise is being able to properly identify specific anatomical structures of the body. The following section contains illustrations and diagrams of the human axial and appendicular skeletal systems and the associated muscular anatomy. As a personal trainer, you will be expected to know the anatomical terms and apply the terms to describe specific body movement.

Procedures
Using the terms provided, correctly label the following anatomical structures. You may refer to Chapter 1 of your course textbook to assist you.

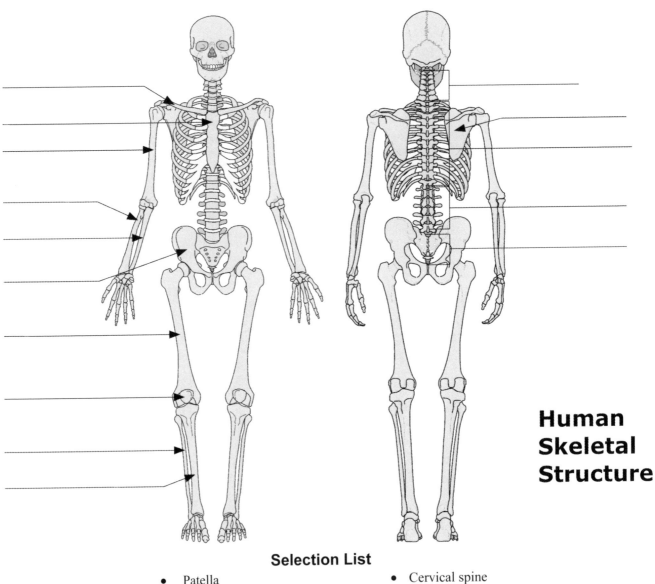

Human Skeletal Structure

Selection List

- Patella
- Radius
- Humerus
- Scapula
- Fibula
- Ulna
- Femur
- Tibia

- Cervical spine
- Thoracic spine
- Lumbar spine
- Pelvis
- Clavicle
- Sacrum & Coccyx
- Sternum

Upper Body Anterior View

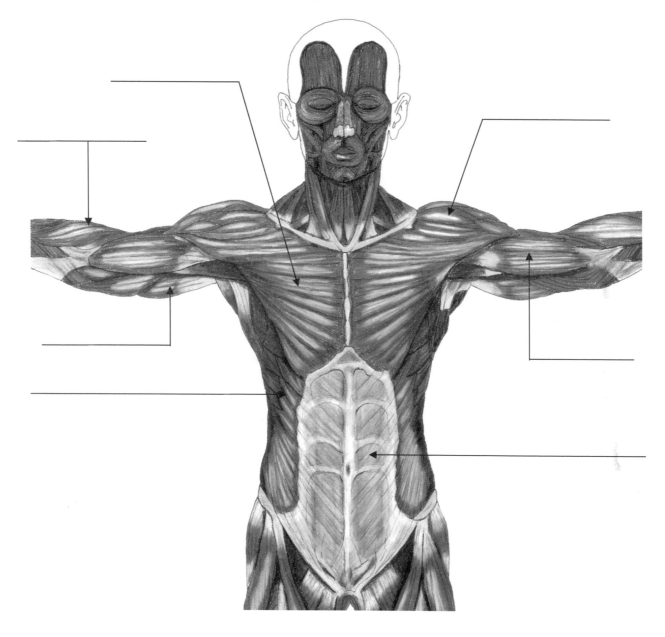

Selection List

- Rectus Abdominis
- Pectoralis Major
- Triceps Brachii
- Deltoid
- Biceps Brachii
- Brachioradialis
- External Oblique

Upper Body Posterior View

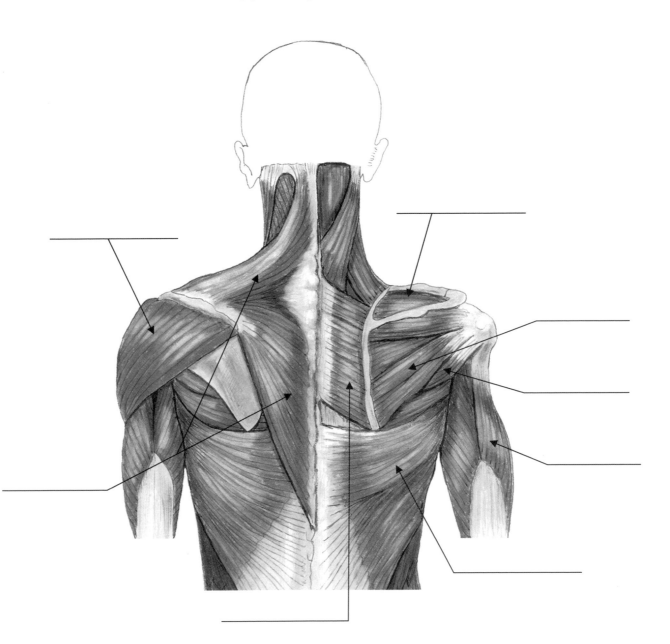

Selection List

- Teres Minor
- Infraspinatus
- Supraspinatus
- Deltoid

- Trapezius
- Latissimus Dorsi
- Tricep Brachii
- Rhomboid Major

Lower Body Anterior View

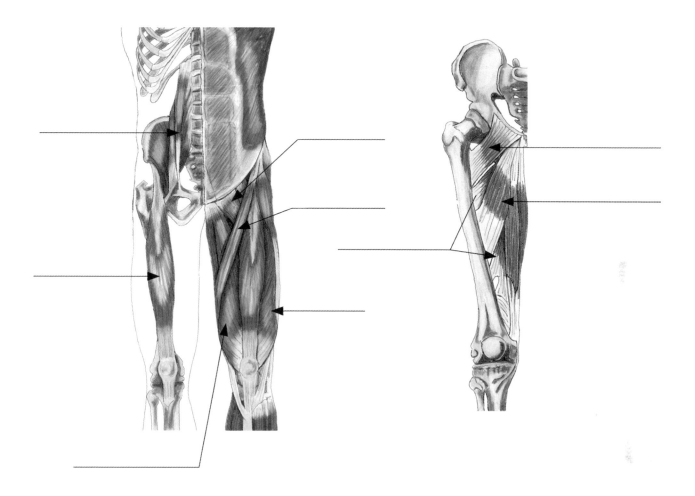

Selection List

- Psoas Major
- Rectus Femoris
- Vastus Medialis
- Pectineus
- Sartorius

- Vastus Lateralis
- Adductor Magnus
- Adductor Longus
- Adductor Brevis

Lower Body Posterior View

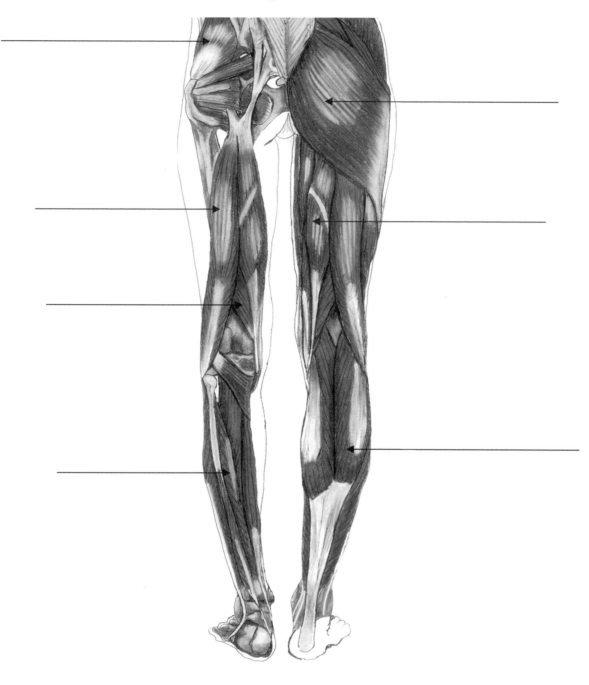

Selection List

- Gluteus Medius
- Gluteus Maximus
- Semitendinosus
- Biceps Femoris
- Semimembranosus
- Soleus
- Gastrocnemius

Procedures

Identify the muscle cell structures by filling in the spaces provided. Select the answers from the list of terms provided below. You may refer to Chapter 3 of your course textbook to assist you.

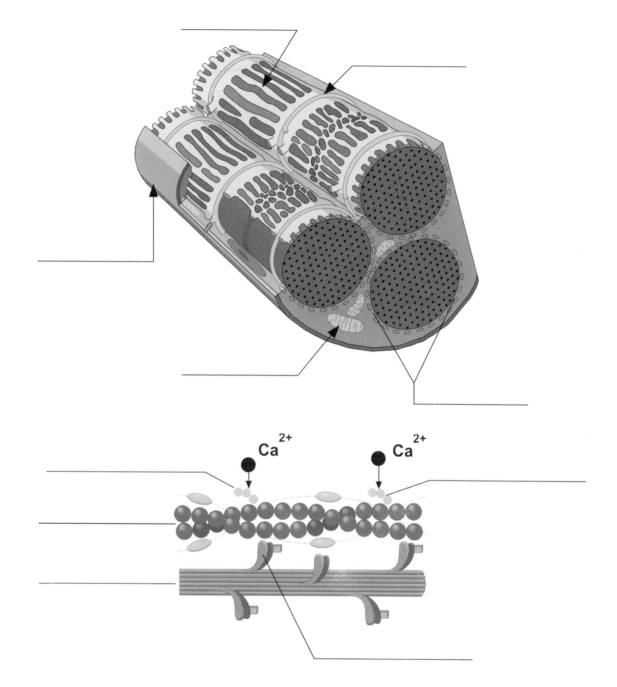

Selection List

- Troponin (Two Locations)
- Myosin
- Actin
- Crossbridges
- T-tubules

- Mitochondria
- Myofibril
- Sarcoplasmic Reticulum
- Muscle Fascia

Match the identified structure from the previous selection list with its respective role in a muscle contraction.

1. _____ is the thin myofilament used during muscle contractions.

2. _____ contain contractile elements which generate tension during a muscle contraction.

3. _____ stores and releases calcium when stimulated by an action potential.

4. _____ is used as a shuttle system for myofibrillar activity.

5. _____ contains enzymes used for aerobic metabolism in the cell.

6. _____ is the heavy chain contractile element found within the sarcomere.

Activity 1.2 Movement Description

Activity Description

Anatomists have developed a vocabulary to describe specific anatomical movements, identify the position of specific anatomical structures, describe muscle function as it relates to movement, and describe different types of muscle contractions. The terms, which are listed and categorized under this activity, are widely employed in the exercise science and fitness training environments. It is important that you become familiar with the working definitions of these terms, particularly as they relate to human movement and exercise.

Procedures

In the spaces provided identify and label the pelvic position demonstrated in the illustrations below.

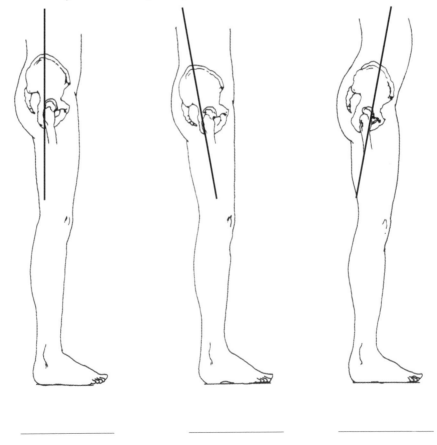

_____   _____   _____

Procedures

Identify the pelvic position used for the following exercises. Choose from one of the following pelvic positions: Anterior Pelvic Tilt, Posterior Pelvic Tilt, and Neutral Pelvic Tilt.

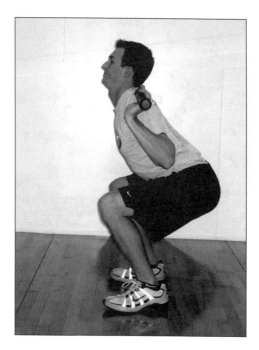

Pelvic Position:_____

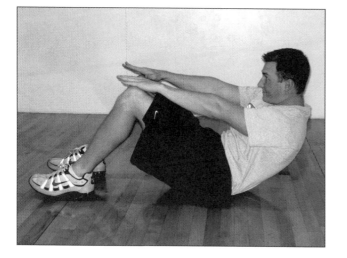

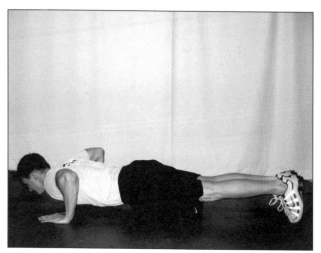

Pelvic Position:_____   Pelvic Position:_____

Procedures

Identify the joint actions and muscle groups involved in the following exercises. Each action performed by the body during the execution of the movement should be included in the spaces provided. The joint movements and muscle groups should be selected from the lists provided. The exercises can be referenced in Chapter 19 of the course textbook.

Selection List

Movement		Muscles and Muscle Groups	
Elevation	Depression	Quadriceps	Hamstrings
Protraction	Retraction	Gastrocnemius	Soleus
Abduction	Adduction	Hip Adductors	Hip Abductors
Horizontal Abduction	Horizontal Adduction	Iliopsoas	Back Extensors
Internal Rotation	External Rotation	Gluteals	Latissimus Dorsi
Flexion	Extension	Rhomboids	Trapezius
Hyperextension	Pronation	Deltoids	Rotator Cuff
Supination		Pectoralis Major	Lateral Obliques
		Rectus Abdominis	Biceps
		Triceps	Brachioradialis

Fill in the blanks for each exercise

1. **Exercise Name:** <u>Abdominal Crunch</u>

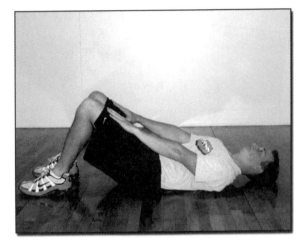
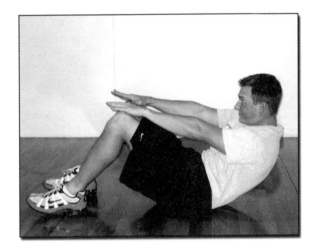

Starting Position   Ending Position

Joint Action(s): _____

Muscle(s) involved: _____

2. **Exercise Name:** Tricep Extension

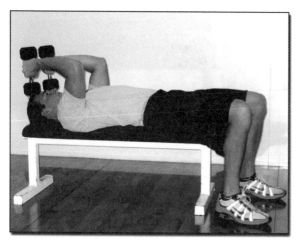   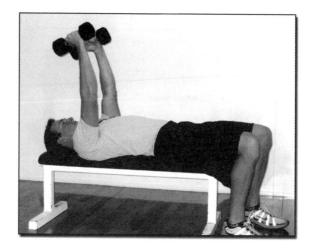

Starting Position   Ending Position

Joint Action(s): _____

Muscle(s) involved: _____

3. **Exercise Name:** Step-up

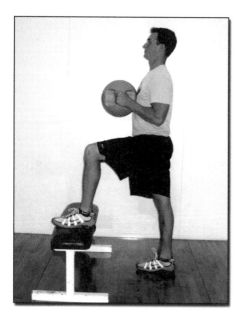   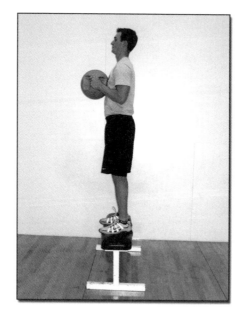

Starting Position   Ending Position

Joint Action(s): _____

Muscle(s) involved: _____

4. **Exercise Name:** <u>Bench Push-up</u>

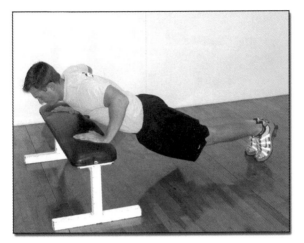

Starting Position

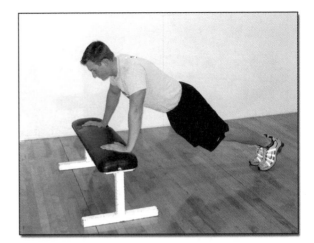

Ending Position

Joint Action(s): _____

Muscle(s) involved: _____

5. **Exercise Name:** <u>Squat</u>

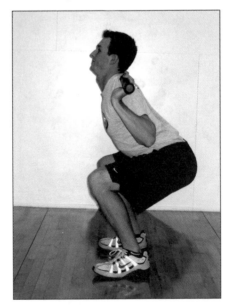

Starting Position

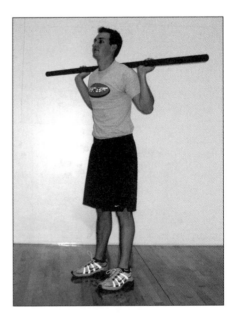

Ending Position

Joint Action(s): _____

Muscle(s) involved: _____

6. **Exercise Name:** <u>Seated Row</u>

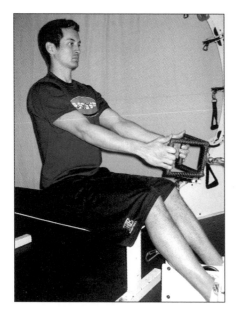

Starting Position

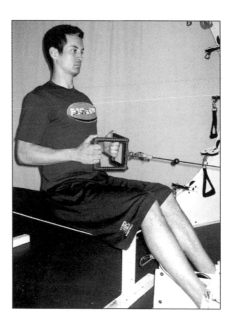

Ending Position

Joint Action(s): _____

Muscle(s) involved: _____

7. **Exercise Name:** <u>Romanian Deadlift</u>

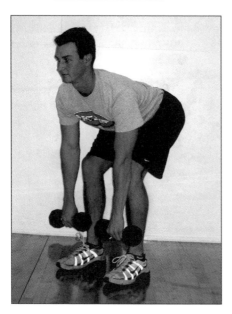

Starting Position

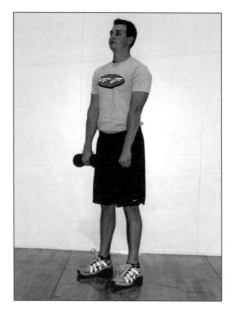

Ending Position

Joint Action(s): _____

Muscle(s) involved: _____

8. Exercise Name: <u>Lunge</u>

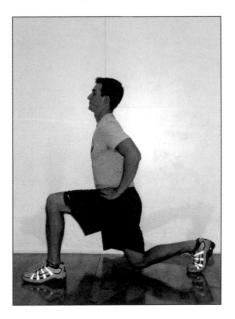

Starting Position   Ending Position

Joint Action(s): _____

Muscle(s) involved: _____

Activity 1.3 Anatomical Planes
Activity Description

Once the structures of the body can be identified and a working knowledge of the previous anatomical terms has been established, the terms can be applied to the planes of movement. This will allow for a complete description of any number of actions.

An anatomical plane is an imaginary, flat, two-dimensional surface that divides the body into various segments. Anatomical planes describe positions, relationships, and directions of movement by, and within the human body.

Procedures

Fill in the appropriate plane in the spaces provided. You can refer to Chapter 1 of your textbook for assistance.

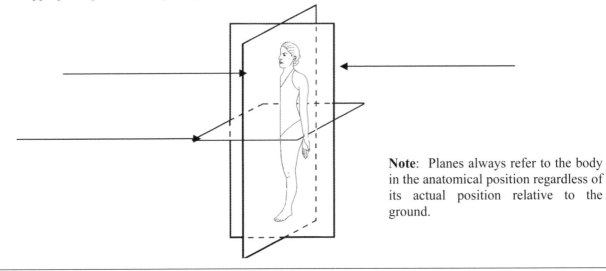

Note: Planes always refer to the body in the anatomical position regardless of its actual position relative to the ground.

Procedures

Identify the joint action and plane of movement used during each of the following exercises. If more than one plane is used identify the individual joint structure and its respective movement plane.

1. **Exercise Name:** <u>Dumbbell Chest Press</u>

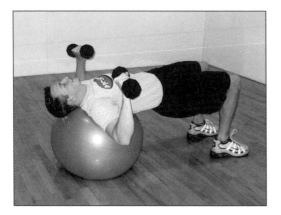 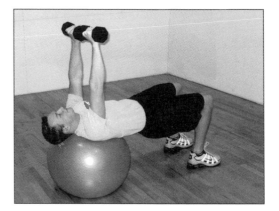

Joint Action(s):_____

Movement Plane(s):_____

2. **Exercise Name:** <u>Lat Pull-down</u>

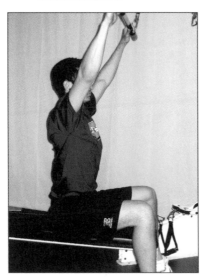 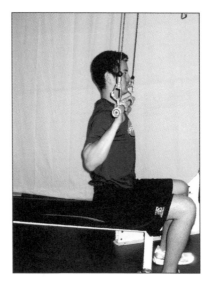

Joint Action(s):_____

Movement Plane(s):_____

3. **Exercise Name:** <u>Lunge with Rotation</u>

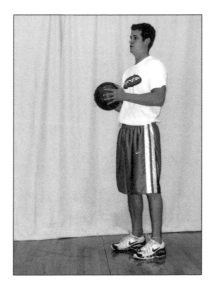 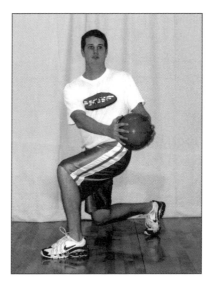

Joint Action(s):_____

Movement Plane(s):_____

4. **Exercise Name:** <u>Diagonal Chop on Physioball</u>

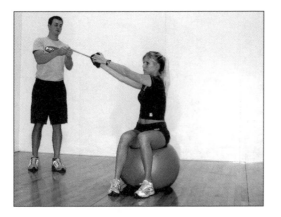 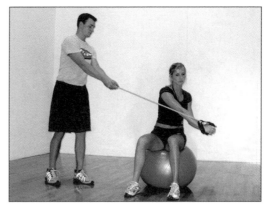

Joint Action(s):_____

Movement Plane(s):_____

Activity 1.4 Understanding Stability

Activity Description

Basic motor control is a factor of maintaining one's balance under varying applications of force from different directions. The ability to stabilize a joint or group of joints to successfully perform a movement or maintain balance is an important consideration for exercise selection. Three critical factors that affect the stability of an object include the size of the base of support, the relation of the line of gravity to the base of support, and the location or height of the center of gravity. Exercises can be modified to become more or less challenging by manipulating these factors.

Procedures

Order the exercises by their relative stability requirements from easiest to perform to the most difficult assuming each exercise is performed at the same level of intensity and for the same duration. Justify your answer using the basic principles of stability found in Chapter 2 of your course textbook. Illustrations of these movements can be found in Chapter 19 of your course textbook.

Group One

_____ Bench press

_____ Physioball push-up

_____ Standing band press

Explanation:_____

Group Two

_____ Bent-over row

_____ Seated row

_____ Lat pull-down

Explanation:_____

Group Three

_____ Deadlift

_____ Back squat

_____ Leg press

Explanation:_____

Group Four

_____ Side raise

_____ Seated dumbbell press

_____ Front raise

Explanation:_____

Lab I Submission Form – Functional Movement Applications

1. Which muscle of the quadriceps crosses both the knee and hip joint playing a role in both knee extension and hip flexion? _____ .

2. Complete the following sentences using the proper terminology or muscle.

    The quadriceps are _____ contracted during the downward phase of the deadlift exercise.

    The abdominals are contracted _____ during the standing military press.

    The agonist muscle during the bent-over row is the _____.

    The antagonist muscle in the back extension exercise is the _____.

    The prime mover for the back squat exercise is the _____.

3. If the crest of the pelvis moves forward and down, the pelvis is said to be in a(n) _____ pelvic tilt.

4. Which type of pelvic tilt should precede abdominal exercises in the supine position?

    _____

5. Identify the muscle(s) that perform the functions listed:

Name of Muscle	Primary Function
_____	Internal Trunk Rotation
_____	Shoulder Adduction
_____	Hip Flexion
_____	Knee Flexion

6. List the three factors that affect the stability of an exercise.

    1. _____

    2. _____

    3. _____

Lab I Submission Form – Functional Movement Applications

7. Identify the plane of movement used for each of the following exercises.

Lateral Raise: _____

Abdominal Curl-up: _____

Medicine Ball Torso Twist:_____

Reverse Lunge: _____

8. Identify the primary joint movements of the following exercises.

Lat Pull-down: _____

Bench Press: _____

Shoulder Press: _____

9. Identify the bone found at each location.

Thigh: _____

Upper Arm: _____

10. Identify the muscles that make up the hamstring muscle group.

_____

_____

_____

Lab Two
Energy Systems, Hormones, and the Heart

Lab Two corresponds to the following textbook readings:

Endocrine System	Chapter 4
Bioenergetics	Chapter 5
Cardiovascular Physiology	Chapter 6

Lab Description
Lab Two is designed to expose students to the physiological systems of the body that function to support exercise. The first section identifies the hormones that support exercise and contribute to the adaptation response to varying physical stress. Section two identifies the energy pathways that support physical activity and the resultant internal activities that necessitate recovery from physical stress. Section three covers the function of the heart and resting measures that indicate the health and efficiency of the cardiovascular system.

Explored Procedures
- Identification of Hormones and their Function
- Energy System Interaction
- Energy System Contribution – Box Step
- Myocardium Structural Identification
- Resting Heart Rate Assessment and Evaluation
- Resting Blood Pressure Assessment and Evaluation

Lab Objectives
- Identify the hormonal responses to stress and exercise
- Identify the energy systems that drive anaerobic and aerobic exercise
- Explain the interaction of energy systems during low and high intensity activity
- Accurately identify important myocardial structures/landmarks
- Explain the blood flow pattern of the heart
- Identify and explain the mechanisms that control heart rate and heart rate responses
- Understand the physiological significance of resting heart rate values and specific training adaptations
- Successfully palpate a subject's carotid and radial pulse to determine resting heart rate
- Successfully administer a resting blood pressure assessment
- Identify and explain the mechanisms that control blood pressure and blood pressure responses
- Understand the physiological significance of resting blood pressure values and specific training adaptations that affect it

Activity 2.1 Hormonal Activity
Activity Description
In addition to the maintenance of physiological homeostasis, the endocrine system is used to manage physical and psychological stress response. Training response is indicative of the stress experienced by the body, as are the resultant adaptations to the perceived stress. Hormones serve as chemical messengers between endocrine glands and tissues and target cells, dictating specific actions. Understanding the relationship between physical activity, hormonal response, and resultant adaptations are integral to exercise programming.

Procedures

For each hormone provided, identify where it is produced, the function of the hormone, and the stimulus associated with its release. Chapter 4 of your textbook may be referenced for assistance if necessary.

Testosterone

Gland: _____

Function: _____

Stimulus for Release: _____

Physiological Effects: _____

Human Growth Hormone

Gland: _____

Function: _____

Stimulus for Release: _____

Physiological Effects: _____

Thyroxine (T-3, T-4)

Gland: _____

Function: _____

Stimulus for Release: _____

Physiological Effects: _____

Insulin-like Growth Factor

Gland: _____

Function: _____

Stimulus for Release: _____

Physiological Effects: _____

Cortisol

Gland: _____

Function: _____

Stimulus for Release: _____

Physiological Effects: _____

Epinephrine

Gland: _____

Function: _____

Stimulus for Release: _____

Physiological Effects: _____

Norepinephrine

Gland: _____

Function: _____

Stimulus for Release: _____

Physiological Effects: _____

Activity 2.2 Anaerobic Power Step Test

Activity Description

The metabolic systems of the body are designed to meet specific demands. The duration of time and intensity by which the activity is performed ultimately determines the energy system contribution. When the intensity is elevated and prolonged, the different energy systems attempt to maximize the ATP production to support the force output requirements, but each system has limits to its ATP production.

The anaerobic power step forces the body to move through the phosphagen system and into glycolytic pathways. The decline in force output can be tracked by identifying the shifts in contribution from each system. The assessment lasts for 60 seconds, which enables it to measure both short and long-term anaerobic power. The energy requirement is primarily dependent upon the glycolytic pathway of anaerobic metabolism with secondary support from the phosphagen energy system. Due to the length of the test and the intensity at which it is performed, a high amount of lactic acid can be expected. It is somewhat isolated from the general circulation because only one leg is used for the test. The test is an excellent example of the body's response to high intensity anaerobic training reflected by a decline in movement speed, increased heart rate, and respiration rate in response to changing pH levels.

Equipment
Step or box
Stopwatch

Procedures

Step 1   **Start Position**: The subject should stand alongside a box or bench. The height of the bench should allow the knee to be flexed at 90 degrees.

Step 2   The subject starts with the foot of their dominant leg (testing leg) centered on top of the box or bench. The step foot will remain in the same location throughout the duration of the test.

Step 3   **Start Test**: On the "Go" command, the trainer starts the timer and the subject begins the step-up. On each step, the subject's legs and back should be straightened with the arms remaining at the sides of the body being used for balance only. The arms should not move for the purpose of momentum assistance.

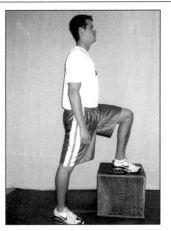 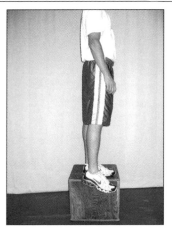

Step 4   The cadence for the test is a 1-2 count; the 1 count is up and the 2 count is down. Tests should not be paced, but performed at an all-out exertion for the entire duration (60 seconds).

Step 5   **Scoring**: A step is counted each time the subject's step leg is straightened and then returned to the starting position. Steps are not counted if the subject does not straighten the step leg or if the subject's back is bent.

Step 6   The trainer should call out the time remaining every 15 seconds. The total number of steps should be recorded for the sixty second trial.

Step 7   **Stop Test**: At the end of the 60 second period, the trainer should stop the test and record the number of steps.

Number of Steps Completed _____

Step 8   Have the subject perform a cool down to prevent blood pooling in the action leg.

How to Calculate

Anaerobic Capacity (kgm · min^{-1}) = {_____ kg x [(0.4 m x _____ step score)/1]} x 1.33

$$= [_____ \text{ kg x } (_____) \text{ m } / 1] \text{ x } 1.33$$

$$= _____ \text{ kg x } _____ \text{m} \cdot \text{min}^{-1} \text{ x } 1.33$$

$$= _____ (\text{kgm} \cdot \text{min}^{-1})$$

Watts $= _____ (\text{kgm} \cdot \text{min}^{-1}) \div 6.12 \text{ W/ kgm} \cdot \text{m}^{-1}$

Example

A 100 kg (220 lb) male completed 60 steps for the entire one minute test duration.

Anaerobic Capacity (kgm · min^{-1}) = 100 x [(0.40 x 60)/1] x 1.33

= [100 x (24/1)] x1.33

= 100 x 24.0 x 1.33

= 3192 (kgm · min^{-1})

Conversion to Watts (6.12 kgm · min^{-1} = 1 W)

Watts = 3192 ÷ 6.12

= 521.6 W

Classification for Anaerobic Capacity		
	Male Power (W)	Female Power (W)
Above Average	≥507	≥339
Average	460-506	307-338
Below Average	<460	<307

Activity 2.3 Energy Systems

Procedures

Aerobic and anaerobic energy systems support physical activities based on the duration of time and intensity of the work performed. Identify the primary energy system used for each activity. Select from the list provided. Reference Chapter 5 in your textbook for assistance if needed.

Selection List
ATP
Creatine Phosphate
Anaerobic Glycolysis
Aerobic Metabolism

1. 3RM Squat: _____

2. 5 Minute Jump Rope: _____

3. 100 Meter Sprint: _____

4. Vertical Jump: _____

5. 10RM Leg Press: _____

6. 20 Minutes Interval Training: _____

7. 30 Minute Steady-state Jog: _____

Activity 2.4 Myocardial Structural Identification & Blood Flow

Activity Description

The cardiac muscle, also known as the myocardium, is the most important muscle in the body. Like the other muscles of the body, the myocardium experiences significant changes when stress is applied through exercise. The heart is a four-chambered dual pump system responsible for circulating oxygenated blood throughout the body. The average healthy heart circulates over 1,900 gallons of blood per day. It is a very efficient muscle and contains an extraordinary amount of mitochondria to quickly meet the changing oxygen demands of the cardiac tissue. In fact, cardiac muscle has a 50% greater ability to extract oxygen than voluntary striated muscle making it more suited for its endurance need.

Procedures
Using the provided terms, properly label the following cardiac structures.

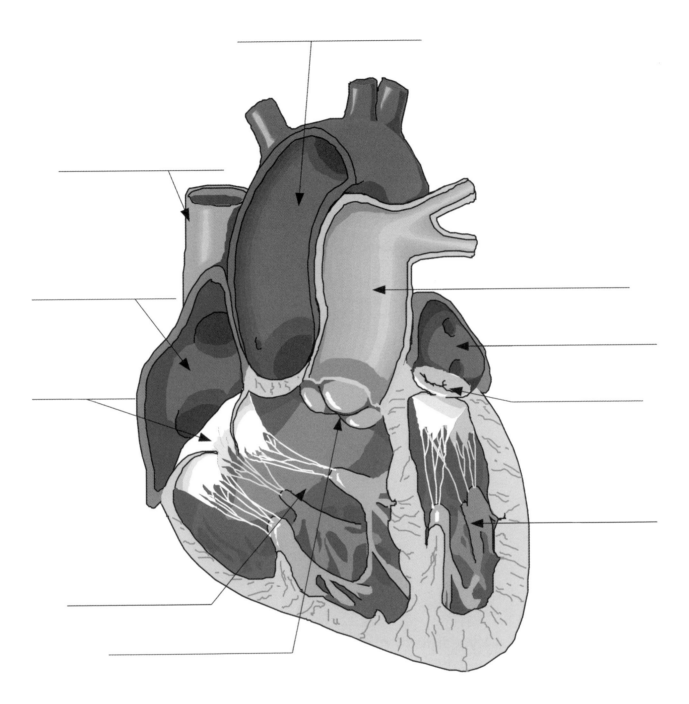

Selection List

Aorta   Left Atrium
Left Ventricle   Right Ventricle
Superior Vena Cava   Bicuspid Valve
Pulmonary Artery   Pulmonary Semilunar Valve
Tricuspid Valve   Right Atrium

Procedures

Identify the path of blood flow through the heart using the appropriate spaces in the text. Select from the list provided.

Blood Flow Through the Heart

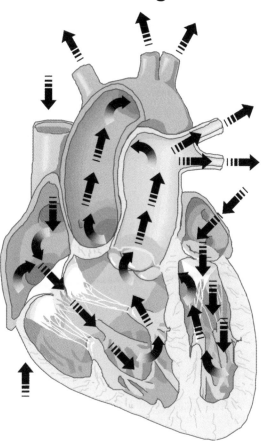

Selection List

Left Ventricle
Right Ventricle
Aorta
Pulmonary Artery
Pulmonary Vein
Left Atrium
Right Atrium

The blood enters the heart from venous circulation into the _____. It is pumped through the

tricuspid valve into the _____. Upon contraction, the tricuspid valve is forced shut and the blood is

pumped through the pulmonary semilunar valve into the _____. The blood is oxygenated at the lungs

and is transferred back to the heart through the _____ where it enters the _____.

The blood is then pumped through the bicuspid valve into the _____. Upon contraction, the blood is

forced through the aortic valve into the _____ entering arterial circulation.

Resting Cardiovascular Measurements

The two most common cardiovascular parameters assessed by fitness professionals are heart rate and blood pressure. These measurements are valuable in identifying warning signs and physical indications of what is occurring within the body. They serve as a vital part of the entire screening and evaluation segment of a client's profile. Due to the fact that both the parasympathetic and sympathetic nervous systems control cardiovascular responses, even simple psychological stress can activate a change in resting cardiovascular activity. Developing a clear understanding as to the cause and effect phenomenon will help you identify factors that should be addressed to reduce risk for disease and move toward optimal health attainment.

Fitness professionals are expected to properly perform these vital assessments on their clients, as necessary, to carry out professional responsibilities. The results from these physical assessments are used to: clear a client for entry into an exercise program; establish baseline measurements by which future assessments can be compared for monitoring program effectiveness; identify possible health risks; assist in establishment of cardiovascular training zones; provide limited insight into a client's current psychological and physiological state; and provide the client with pertinent information regarding his or her health status based on population norms and mortality rates.

Resting Heart Rate

At rest, heart rate is subject to mild changes influenced by such factors as state of arousal, posture, hormones, and other bio-chemically related phenomenon. Resting heart rate, even under conditions of mild stress, is restrained by action of the vagus nerve. Vagal tone describes the level of restraint applied to the myocardium and is elevated at rest. This means a decrease of roughly 10 to 15 beats per minute. During exercise, vagal tone is released as sympathetic stimulation increases and mechanical receptors influence the speed of the heart's contractions. Even with the natural defense mechanism action of the vagus nerve, heart rate will still increase based upon constant agitators. Additional stress to the body will influence heart rate variance when the stress is constantly applied to the body. Common examples of chronic stress factors include excess fat weight, Type A personality, work related or emotional stress, and reduced oxygen availability from smoking or the environment. However, the increased heart rate caused by these stressors does not provide the positive physiological adaptation responses seen with exercise aimed at heart rate elevation. They rather serve as a form of distress, which can eventually manifest into disease.

Sedentary or deconditioned individuals experience greater heart rate requirements both at rest and during exercise due to their lack of cardiorespiratory efficiency. Trained individuals have much stronger hearts, evidenced by higher stroke volumes (expulsion of blood from the left ventricle of the heart per beat) and can expel greater quantities of blood with better economy. They are afforded less heart rate requirements because they have a better pump mechanism. Therefore, a lower resting heart rate is indicative of someone who is in better cardiovascular condition. Conversely, someone with an elevated resting heart rate is subject to greater health risks. For this reason, elevated resting heart rates require specific attention, and a medical referral is required for individuals with a pulse equal to, or greater than 100 beats • min⁻¹.

Resting Blood Pressure

The other important resting physiological measurement assessed by the fitness professional during the initial screening process is blood pressure. Resting blood pressure is influenced by a number of factors and it alone can be a strong indicator of cardiovascular health. As with resting heart rate, the evaluation of blood pressure is a non-invasive measurement, which provides information as to the overall efficiency of the cardiovascular system to deliver blood throughout the body.

Blood pressure is characterized by two values expressed as mmHg (millimeters of mercury as seen in a mercury manometer). The top value reflects the amount of vascular pressure experienced during left ventricular contraction, or systole. It is called systolic blood pressure (SBP). SBP is affected by a number of factors including cardiac output, peripheral resistance, and arterial elasticity. At rest, this value should be around 120 mmHg, although variations in both directions do occur. Heavily muscled individuals will often show an elevation of mercury above the 120 mmHg mark due to additional compression forces upon the vessels, whereas smaller females may have a systolic blood pressure below 110 mmHg due to their smaller heart size.

When the heart enters the relaxation phase of the cardiac cycle, or diastole, the arterial pressure is dramatically decreased. The value then indicates the amount of peripheral resistance within the vessels. A common or normal resting measurement of diastolic blood pressure is 80 mmHg. When this measure is high it indicates that the pressure within the arteries is not dissipating quickly, suggesting slow movement of the blood from the arterioles into the capillaries. This may be due to decreased elasticity in the vessel wall and/or increased peripheral resistance. A systolic pressure of >160 mmHg or a diastolic pressure of >100 mmHg requires a medical referral prior to an individual engaging in physical activity.

As mentioned earlier, resting measurements are subject to external and internal factors. When clients are being assessed, there are conditions and stimuli that can cause a false positive or variations within the measurement. White coat syndrome is one of the more recognized conditions that cause a false positive or artificial rise in HR and BP. It is characterized by an elevation of one or both of these measurements due to a subject's elevated anxiety levels in response to being evaluated (as in the case of a medical evaluation from a physician).

In addition to the above, chemicals and their mediators dictate an aspect of the physiological environment. Consumption of caffeine and other stimulants can elevate resting cardiovascular readings due to their excitation effect on the sympathetic nervous system. Conversely, some classifications of medications will depress the responses of the sympathetic nervous system, particularly with regard to heart rate and blood pressure responses. When working with clients it is important to understand how these factors affect assessment outcomes; dictate health responses; provide insight into the current health level; and direct program classification, admittance, and guidelines.

Hypertension is the most common form of cardiovascular disease. It is characterized by a blood pressure reading of greater than or equal to 140/90 mmHg. If either measurement is over the borderline values of 140/90 mmHg the subject is said to have hypertension. As mentioned earlier, blood pressure readings of 160/100 mmHg or higher necessitates a medical referral for clearance into an exercise program.

Due to the fact that hypertension has been associated with elevated risk of cardiovascular disease, the need for regular monitoring and maintenance of healthy blood pressure is apparent. As a fitness professional performing a thorough screening analysis of a new client, you may identify a person's hypertensive condition and must refer them for further medical diagnosis and care. It is the responsibility of a competent trainer not only to regularly monitor a client's blood pressure, particularly those at risk, but to educate the client as to what blood pressure is and the risks involved with high levels.

Activity 2.5 Administration of Resting Heart Rate

Activity Description

Fitness professionals are often required to assess client heart rate through the manual palpation method. Palpation simply refers to using the sense of touch to monitor or assess a physiological variable or structure of the body. Pulses are generated from the whip-like action of the aorta, whereas the vibration pulse (apical beat) is generated by the left ventricle hitting against the chest wall near the 5th rib. The arterial pulses that may be located and assessed most easily are the radial, carotid, and temporal. In most cases, fitness professionals use the radial pulse for assessment.

The common carotid artery sites are located on both sides of the frontal aspect of the neck. Each is found in the groove formed by the larynx and the sternocleidomastoid muscles just below the mandible. The carotid pulse is taken by placing the first two fingers of the hand in the groove and gently pressing inward. You will feel the pulse immediately if the location site is correct. There has been some evidence to suggest that the pressure exerted from the palpation of this site may cause the baroreceptors in the carotid sinus to cause a temporary decreased heart rate response in some individuals. For this reason it is recommended to wait a few seconds when assessing the pulse before starting the count. Additionally, caution should be taken not to press too hard against the artery as the possibility of fainting or lightheadedness may result. This is of most concern in post exercise assessment.

Palpation of the radial artery is done by placing the first two fingers near the distal end of the radius, just below the base of the thumb. This is the location where the normally deep-running radial artery travels superficially into the hand. By placing the first two fingers over this region and gently pressing, the radial pulse can be palpated. There may be some difficulty locating this pulse in individuals who have large amounts of subcutaneous fat, a weak pulse, or deep-lying vessels. In cases such as these, the carotid pulse may better serve as the palpation site. The thumb should <u>not</u> be used to palpate a subject's pulse because it has a pulse of its own which may interfere with the proper palpation of the site.

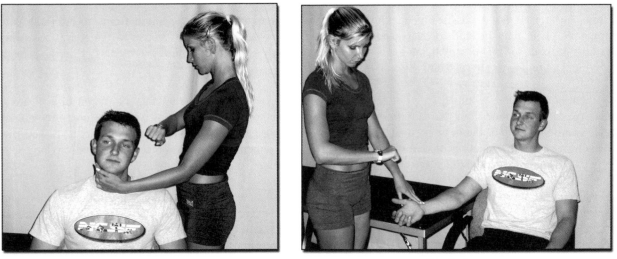

Carotid   **Radial**

The length of time a pulse is taken is dependent on the purpose of the administration and the accuracy required. A pulse count that is taken for only 6 seconds may have a larger degree of error than one that is taken for 30 seconds or a full minute due to possible tester error and pulse deviations. For accurate resting pulse counts, the NCSF recommends taking the pulse for 60 seconds to determine the subject's <u>resting</u> heart rate in beats • min $^{-1}$. During exercise, smaller time increments are used to assess the subject's heart rate, usually 10 or 15 second counts.

Procedures
Using the guidelines below, administer a resting heart rate assessment on a volunteer.

Step 1   Administration of any resting physiological parameter requires the subject to be in a relaxed seated position with both feet flat on the floor. He or she should refrain from any activity for a minimum of 10 minutes prior to measuring resting heart rate. This will ensure that the heart rate is at a true resting state.

Step 2   Ask the subject if they have consumed any stimulants such as caffeine or nicotine, or if they have taken any medications prior to the evaluation, as this may affect resting values.

Step 3   Following the aforementioned palpation protocols, administer a 30 second and 60 second resting heart rate assessment on a volunteer subject using both the brachial and carotid palpation sites. As you palpate your lab partner's pulse, the lab partner should palpate his or her own pulse using the other palpation site. This will aid in accuracy and increase experience at palpating different sites. At the conclusion of the predetermined evaluation period the tester and subject should compare values to ensure that the tester and subject are accurately monitoring the correct pulse count.

Step 4   Record the heart rate values in the spaces provided and compare your results to the norms for resting heart rate.

30 second pulse count

_____ beats x 2 = _____ beats • min $^{-1}$

60 second pulse count

_____ beats • min $^{-1}$

Resting Heart Rate in Men and Women (beats/min)

%	MEN					WOMEN				
	20-29 y	30-39 y	40-49 y	50-59 y	60+ y	20-29 y	30-39 y	40-49 y	50-59 y	60+ y
90	50	50	50	50	52	55	55	55	55	52
80	54	55	54	55	55	59	58	60	60	57
70	58	58	58	58	58	60	62	62	61	60
60	60	60	60	60	60	63	65	64	64	62
50	63	63	62	63	62	65	68	66	67	64
40	66	65	65	65	65	70	70	70	69	66
30	70	68	69	68	68	72	74	72	72	72
20	72	72	72	72	72	75	76	76	75	74
10	80	77	78	77	77	84	82	80	83	79

Data from the US Department of Health and Human Services

Activity 2.6 Administration of Resting Blood Pressure

Activity Description

Blood pressure (BP) is a product of cardiac output (heart rate · stroke volume) and the total peripheral resistance which is measured in mmHg. The administration of a blood pressure evaluation procedure prior to beginning a fitness exercise program will assist the fitness professional in making physical activity inclusion decisions for the client; identify a possible hypertensive condition requiring medical referral; establish a baseline value to which future assessment comparisons can be made; and provide the client with valuable information pertaining to health status as it relates to blood pressure.

There are several non-invasive tools available to the fitness professional to assess and monitor a client's blood pressure. These require the use of a sphygmomanometer (pronounced sfig-mo-ma-nom-e-ter) or commonly referred to as a manometer. Manometers are available in several types, from mercury or needle gauge to electronic measuring instruments. These devices measure the blood pressure in millimeters of mercury (mmHg). This lab will present general guidelines for the administration of a resting blood pressure assessment using a cuff manometer. Individual administration protocols are determined by the device used (digital, mercury, aneroid, etc.) It is recommended that you become proficient using several types of manometers as future work environments may have different measuring devices or protocol requirements.

It is also important to note that if an individual's first assessment is elevated above acceptable guidelines or previously established values, one should repeat the assessment again after a few minutes. The white coat syndrome (explained earlier) may adversely affect readings and/or the subject may need more time to relax in a comfortable seated position.

Procedures

Blood pressure assessments, as with most fitness related assessments, take a large amount of practice in order to become proficient in the execution of the measurement. Use a volunteer subject to accurately assess blood pressure while adhering to the following administration procedures.

Activity Equipment

- Sphygmomanometer (cuff manometer)
    - Mercury or
    - Aneroid or
    - Electronic/digital
- Stethoscope – to auscultate the Korotkoff sound when using a manual cuff manometer
- Tape measure

Step 1   *Select Cuff Size.* There are several cuff sizes available for the manometers. Measure the resting arm circumference of your subject using a metric measuring tape. The following chart will assist you in identifying the correct cuff size for the evaluation (1 inch = 2.54 cm).

Upper Arm Circumference (cm)	Type of Cuff	Bladder Size (cm)
33-47	Large Adult	33 or 42 x 15
25-35	Adult	24 x 12.5
18-26	Child	21.5 x 10

An improper fitting cuff may provide the user with false information. Using a cuff that is too small may overestimate blood pressure, whereas cuffs that are too large may underestimate blood pressure.

Step 2   *Subject Preparation.* Certain preparation procedures should be followed prior to the administration of any resting physiological assessment. In addition to the normal preparation instruction for the administration of resting heart rate assessment, it is extremely important to give your subject at least five minutes to relax in a comfortable environment prior to the blood pressure measurement or re-measurement. Sleeveless shirts, blouses, or loose fitting sleeves are recommended as the cuff should be in contact with the skin to increase testing accuracy. If the sleeve appears to fit tightly around the subject's arm when rolled up, the shirt should be removed. This will ensure that the artery is not further occluded, which will skew results. The subject should also be in a seated position when the cuff is placed over the arm. This will automatically place the subject's antecubital space at heart level.

Step 3   *Cuff Placement.* There has been much debate over which arm to monitor when assessing the blood pressure of an individual. Researchers recommend that the right arm be used for the assessment. This is partly because of the remote possibility that the genetic anomaly of coarctation between the aorta and subclavian artery will cause an elevated blood pressure and if the pressure is within normal ranges here, it is likely to be normal everywhere.

When placing the cuff over the arm the tester should look for the arterial reference indicator located near the center of the cuff. This should be positioned over the brachial artery. The lower edge of the cuff should be about 1 inch above the antecubital space, which is located on the frontal aspect of the elbow. The brachial artery travels through a groove formed by the bifurcation of the triceps and biceps brachii. If you are using a manual manometer and stethoscope you should locate the artery by palpating the area with the first 2 fingers at the medial antecubital space. This is the location for the head of the stethoscope.

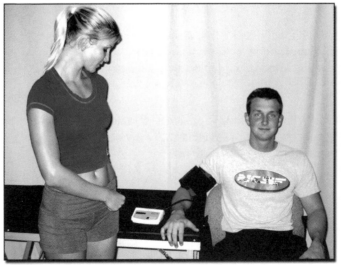

Electronic Manometer

Step 4   *Inflating/Deflating the Cuff.* The determination of blood pressure using the typical manometer device is based upon the sounds made by the vibrations from the vascular walls. These sounds are referred to as Korotkoff sounds (named after their discoverer in 1905). When the cuff is inflated to a predetermined level (see below) the flow of blood through the artery becomes streamlined and the blood begins to "back up" behind the obstruction (in the case of blood pressure reading this will take place on the proximal end of the cuff). As the pressure is released there is a bolus of blood escaping the obstruction and moving through the artery. This bolus of blood causes vascular vibrations that result in a faint sound (systolic pressure reading). As the tester continues to release the air from the bladder more blood escapes through the obstruction caused by the inflated cuff, which causes an even greater vibration and louder sounds heard through the stethoscope. As the pressure is further released from the cuff the blood eventually ceases to vibrate during ventricular contraction. This is due to the lack of obstruction from the decreased pressure placed on the artery from the cuff. The point of the "disappearance of sound" is the diastolic pressure.

Cuff Inflation Pressure(s)

- 160 mmHg females
- 180 mmHg males
- 20 mmHg above expected or known systolic blood pressure
- 30 mmHg above the disappearance of the radial pulse

If you are using an electronic blood pressure device a stethoscope is not needed. The device will assess blood pressure simply by inflating the cuff to a predetermined pressure and then automatically deflate while monitoring systolic and diastolic blood pressures. Most devices will also measure the heart rate of the subject. Typically, the electronic blood pressure devices that assess the brachial artery through the use of a cuff are more accurate than the finger or wrist devices. Be sure to follow manufacturer's directions when using these devices as administration protocols may vary slightly. **Note**: Place the cuff on the subject and position it in the correct location before turning on the electronic device and inflating. The sensors of the cuff will often detect movement and may not provide accurate results if this step is not performed.

Step 5   *Record Results.* Record all results in the spaces provided below. The results will be used to clear a subject for entrance into an exercise program and used for future comparisons

BP 1 _____/_____ mmHg   BP 2 _____/_____ mmHg

Step 6   *Evaluate Results.* The following table contains the gender specific norms for both systolic and diastolic blood pressure. They can be used to help educate your client as to their own health status.

Classification of Blood Pressure for Adults

Blood Pressure Classification	Systolic Blood Pressure (mmHg)	Diastolic Blood Pressure (mmHg)
Normal	<120	And <80
Prehypertension	120-139	Or 80-89
Stage 1 hypertension	140-159	Or 90-99
Stage 2 hypertension	≥160	≥100

Lab Two Submission Form – Energy Systems, Hormones, and the Heart

1. List four anabolic hormones.

   _____

   _____

   _____

   _____

2. List two hormones associated with psychological distress.

   _____

   _____

3. Which chambers of the heart expel blood away from the heart?

   _____ and _____

4. True or false. Arteries contain the majority of the blood in circulation.

5. What resting heart rate response (value) will dictate that the subject needs to seek medical clearance prior to admittance into an exercise program?

   _____ beats • min^{-1}

6. What is the correct course of action if the initial blood pressure for your client is 142/90? Justify your answer.

   _____

   _____

7. The results from a resting heart rate assessment can be used to:

   A._____

   B._____

   C. _____

   D._____

8. What was the resting heart rate and blood pressure of your volunteer subject?

   _____ beats • min^{-1} _____/_____ mmHg

Lab Two Submission Form – Energy Systems, Hormones, and the Heart

9. Hypertension is classified as a blood pressure reading of ≥ _____ mmHg?

10. Ideally, how long should a person remain seated before a resting cardiovascular measurement is performed?

_____

Lab Three
Nutritional Assessment

Lab Three corresponds to the following textbook readings:

Energy Yielding Nutrients	Chapter 7
Non-Energy Yielding Nutrients	Chapter 8
Nutritional Supplementation	Chapter 9

Preface Note: Activity 3.3 of this lab experience requires the student to administer and review a dietary log. It is recommended that each student complete the administration of a dietary food log prior to lab class time so that the analysis can be performed within the lab.

Disclaimer: The information in this lab is intended to provide individuals with information regarding sound nutritional habits and practices. The information is based on the recommendations from the USDA. It is in no way intended to authorize or certify individuals to prescribe specific diets.

Lab Description
The commonality of fad dietary practices and misinformation regarding nutrition and weight loss increases the responsibility of the fitness professional to help disseminate the proper information and assist the client with nutritional education. For all intents and purposes, the concept of short-term "dieting" has not worked, nor will it ever be a stand-alone solution for the achievement of long-term weight goals. Diets have a temporary connotation and the client must understand that for results to be long lasting, their nutritional and physical activity habits must become a normal part of their lifestyle.

A proper diet is one that adequately meets the nutritional needs of the body to support the maintenance, repair, and growth of tissue without providing excess energy that the body stores in the form of adipose tissue. Human nutritional consumption needs are: relative to individual genetic predisposition; affected by normal variations in nutrient digestion, absorption, and assimilation; are needed to meet specific requirements for energy expenditure of physical activity; and influenced by individual dietary preferences. This lends itself to the fact that there is no single diet for optimal nutrition. However, careful evaluation of food consumption, coupled with food intake planning in accordance with sound nutritional guidelines, will result in general and specific improvements in overall health, fitness, and performance.

Explored Procedures
- Reading Food Labels
- Energy Nutrient Intake Requirements
- Implementation of a Food Log
- Dietary Analysis
- Assessment of Hydration Status

Lab Objectives
- Be able to read a food label, analyze its contents, and determine the relevance of the nutrient information
- Be able to establish general energy nutrient needs based on activity status
- Be able to implement and analyze a food log
- Make sound nutritional recommendations based on the RDA's, individual need, and specific training goals
- Analyze hydration replenishment needs based on exercise-related water loss

Activity 3.1 Reading a Food Label

Activity Description

Decisions related to the improvement of a client's dietary behaviors begin with an evaluation of intakes. The first step in the process is learning the difference between portions and serving sizes; an appropriate starting point is teaching the client how to properly read a food label. Although many fitness professionals will opt to utilize one of the many offered nutritional analysis software programs, the information found on labels is relevant when educating clients as to what constitutes good and poor nutritional choices.

Many individuals are directed to follow the recommendations of the DRI-RDA's for energy nutrient consumption. The basic recommendation for caloric intake to reflect ≤30% of total calories from fat, 55%-60% from carbohydrates, and 10%-15% from protein is somewhat difficult to follow based on the fact that computations are necessary to derive these values. Essentially, one must know their total caloric intake, the number of grams of each energy source consumed, and how to covert the numbers into a percentage of total calories. Fitness professionals using these recommendations must first understand how to calculate the percentages and then instruct their clients to be able to do the same. This process all starts with the ability to read a food label.

Procedures

The following food label belongs to a box of macaroni and cheese. For lunch, a 164 lb man prepared the entire box. He consumed ¾ of the box before getting full. Review the label and answer the questions that follow about the nutritional satisfaction of the meal for his daily requirements based on the food label content values for each nutrient (Hint: percentage of calories is calculated by dividing the energy specific calories by total calories).

Nutrition Facts

Serving Size 1 cup
Servings Per Container 4

Amount Per Serving

Calories 230   Calories from Fat 90

	% Daily Value*
Total Fat 10g	13%
Saturated Fat 5g	20%
Cholesterol 24mg	8%
Sodium 730mg	30%
Total Carbohydrates 26g	8%
Dietary Fiber 1g	4%
Sugars 9g	
Protein 9g	

Vitamin A 5%	Vitamin C 0%
Calcium 25%	Iron 6%

Percent Values are based on a 2,000 calorie diet. Your Daily values may be higher or lower depending on your calorie needs:

	Calories	2,000
Total fat		65g
Sat fat		20g
Cholesterol		300mg
Sodium		2,400mg
Total Carbohydrates		300g
Fiber		25g

Calories per gram:
Fat 9   Carbohydrate 4   Protein 4

Answer the following questions related to the food label

1. What is a single serving size? _____ kcal

2. What is the total number of servings reportedly consumed? _____

3. What is the total number of calories consumed by the individual? _____ kcal

4. What percentage of the total calories consumed came from fat? _____ %

5. What percentage of fat calories comes from saturated fat? _____ %

6. What percentage of the total calories consumed came from carbohydrates? _____ %

7. What percentage of the total calories comes from sugars? _____ %

8. How many grams of fiber did this person consume? _____ g

9. What percentage of the total calories consumed came from protein? _____ %

Activity 3.2 Prediction of Energy Yielding Nutrient Requirements
Activity Description
Physical activity is a primary determinant of daily energy requirement. Individual differences exist based on bodyweight, body composition, and the volume of physical activity performed routinely. Individuals who regularly engage in moderate to vigorous exercise and physical activity generally require more calories than comparably sized individuals who are inactive. The determination of specific energy requirements is subject to several factors including the type of activity participated in and the volume and intensity employed on a weekly basis. The following activity identifies general recommendations related to these factors.

Procedures
Using the formulas below calculate the energy intake requirements for each nutrient using yourself or a volunteer subject. The charts can be used to assist in identifying the specific requirements as they relate to individual size and physical activity status.

Carbohydrate Intake

Step 1   Convert bodyweight in pounds into bodyweight in kilograms

Bodyweight _____ lbs.

Bodyweight _____ lbs. ÷ 2.2 = _____ kg

Step 2   Select a carbohydrate intake multiplier from the chart below based on your daily physical activity. If you fall in between whole values you may use a decimal value (example: 4.5 g/kg of bodyweight).

Selected carbohydrate requirement _____ g/kg of bodyweight

Population	Carbohydrate Requirements
Sedentary Individual	3–4 g/kg of bodyweight (BW)
Physically Active	4–5 g/kg of BW
Routine Moderate Exercise	5–6 g/kg of BW
Routine Vigorous Exercise	6–8 g/kg of BW

Step 3   Multiply your weight in kilograms by your selected carbohydrate need.

Weight in kilograms _____ x selected carbohydrate need _____ g/kg = _____ carbohydrate intake requirement in grams

Carbohydrate intake requirement = _____ grams of CHO

Step 4   Multiply your carbohydrate intake requirement by 4 kcal/g carbohydrate to identify the predicted daily caloric intake requirement.

_____ grams of CHO x 4 kcal/g = _____ Daily Carbohydrate Calories

Protein Intake

Step 1   Convert bodyweight in pounds into bodyweight in kilograms

Bodyweight   _____ lbs.

Bodyweight   _____ lbs. ÷ 2.2 = _____ kg

Step 2   Select a protein intake multiplier from the chart below based on your daily physical activity. If you fall in between whole values you may use a decimal value (example: 1.45 g/kg of body weight).

Selected protein requirement _____ g/kg of bodyweight

Population	Protein Intake
Sedentary Individual	0.8 g – 0.9g/kg of bodyweight (BW)
Physically Active	1.0 – 1.2 g/kg of BW
Endurance Athlete	1.3 – 1.5 g/kg of BW
Bodybuilding & Strength Training	1.6 – 2.0 g/kg of BW
Children	Up to 2 g/kg of BW
Pregnant Female	Add 20g to total daily requirements Add 10g if nursing

Step 3   Multiply your weight in kilograms by your selected protein need.

Weight in kilograms _____ x selected protein need _____ g/kg = _____ protein intake requirement in grams

Protein intake requirement = _____ grams of Protein

Step 4   Multiply your protein intake requirement by 4 kcal/g protein to identify the predicted daily caloric intake requirement.

_____ grams of Protein x 4 kcal/g = _____ Daily Protein Calories

Fat Intake

Step 1   Determine your total calories from Carbohydrates and Proteins (CHOPr) by entering your calculated carbohydrate and protein intake from above.

Carbohydrate intake _____ kcal + Protein intake _____ kcal = _____ CHOPr value

Step 2   Select a desired percentage of fat calories from the chart below.

Fat percentage _____ %

Population	Fat Requirements
Sedentary Individual	<30%
Physically Active	25-35%
Obese	*20-25%
High Risk/Disease	*20-25%

Doctor or Registered Dietitian Recommended

Step 3   Complete the formula below by entering your data.

Total calories = (CHOPr value _____ kcal) ÷ {1 - (desired percentage of fat _____ % ÷ 100)}

Total calories = _____

Step 4   Subtract the calculated carbohydrate and protein value (CHOPr value) from the total calories to identify the daily fat calories

Total calories _____ - CHOPr value _____ = _____ kcal from Fat

Predicted daily caloric need based on the sum of the three calculations performed = _____ kcal

Activity 3.3 Nutrition Assessment - 24 Hour Dietary Log/Recall

Activity Description
Note: A 24 hour dietary log needs to be completed prior to this section of the lab.

A dietary log can be very useful in determining the actual amount of energy consumed and the true nutrient content of the diet. It is important to ascertain the nutritional make up of the calories being consumed so that the client is able to meet his or her daily nutritional requirements. Energy nutrient needs will vary depending upon the specific activities the client engages in on a daily basis. The body uses each energy nutrient (fats, proteins, carbohydrates) for specific tasks and therefore must have an ample supply of each nutrient source on a daily basis to meet its biological needs.

The DRI-RDA's provide a recommended intake of energy intended to reflect adequate nutrition for approximately 90% of the population. For physically active individuals variations in energy intakes may be necessary to meet the demands of active lifestyle habits. Individuals who are highly active will not only need more calories to fuel their energy needs, but will need energy specific calories to maximize the performance of the body. Likewise, individuals at high risk for disease may also require modifications to the general recommendations to reduce the risk of further disease progression. Understanding the role of each energy source will better enable the fitness professional to meet the needs of their clients.

To determine shortcomings in the diet and to make appropriate recommendations, the fitness professional must understand how to use dietary logs and be able to implement correct changes to assist in goal attainment. The dietary log allows the fitness professional to take a look into the regular dietary activities of a client and determine what actions need to be taken to intervene in problem eating behaviors. The primary objectives of implementing the dietary log are to:

1. Determine if the caloric needs are adequately being met
2. Analyze the food choices to see if relative nutritional needs are met
3. Assess areas for problems such as lack of nutrient intakes, deficiencies, and risks for disease
4. Identify possible behavior patterns that negatively affect dietary intakes

Administration of a food log to evaluate nutritional intakes is relatively easy. A client is asked to record everything that they consume, including water and all beverages, for a predetermined period of time. Typical dietary logs range in length from 1 to 3 days including at least one weekend day if the dietary log is taken on more than 1 day. Although longer durations are preferred, shorter terms are often more realistic for most people. Some problems to look for and discuss with the client before implementing the dietary log activity include:

- Underreporting – people tend to underestimate or misreport serving sizes or portions
- Vague record keeping – non-specific record keeping provides low quality information
- Temporarily changing eating habits – people modify habits to seem more healthy
- Falsifying data – some individuals become embarrassed about their food consumption

To reduce or minimize these problems, the fitness professional can explain the importance of the assessment and how inaccurate values will affect the client's ability to reach his or her desired goals. It should be made clear that the client will not be criticized or judged for what he or she has consumed. The fitness professional should try to provide the client with models or descriptions of portion sizes (food replicas) and cues to elicit complete detailed responses. In addition, clients should be instructed as to how to read labels and ascertain quantities of foods that are eaten in restaurants and similarly uncontrolled environments. Using photographs of quantified food measures may aid in stimulating recall of consumed portion sizes.

Procedures

Adhering to the following administration protocols, perform a 24-hour dietary log or recall on yourself or a volunteer subject. Upon completion, perform a nutritional assessment using the provided guidelines.

Step 1   If using a volunteer subject, explain the importance of completely and honestly recording all food and drinks consumed. Clearly explain that they should not modify their intake during the assessment. Emphasize that the accuracy and usefulness of the feedback is dependent on the information he or she provides and that they will not be criticized or judged for what they have eaten.

Step 2   Provide measured quantities of common foods the subject may consume so they have a reference for serving sizes. Explain how to use the labels on food products to estimate portion sizes using models and food replicas whenever applicable.

Sample Serving Sizes

Breads, Cereal, Rice, and Pasta Group	Fruit Group	Vegetable Group	Milk, Yogurt, and Cheese Group	Meat, Poultry, Fish, Dry Beans, Eggs, and Nuts Group	Fats, Oils, and Sweets Group
1 slice of bread ½ cup cooked rice or pasta ¾ cup of cereal	1 medium apple, banana, or orange ¾ cup of fruit juice	1 cup raw leafy vegetables ½ cup of cooked carrots or broccoli	1 cup milk or yogurt 1.5 oz natural cheese	2-3 oz cooked lean meat, poultry, or fish 1 cup cooked dry beans	1 T oil 2 T salad dressing 1 T mayonnaise ½ candy bar

Step 3   Provide the following instructions for performance of a 24-hour Recall:

1. Record everything consumed – this includes foods, beverages, and snacks.
2. Record how the food was prepared, being as specific as possible. Any cooking additives must be recorded and amount listed (e.g. 1 T margarine).
3. Indicate the amount of food eaten. Use typical household measures when possible.

    (t = teaspoon, T = tablespoon, c = cup, oz = ounce)

4. Provide brand names and label information when available.
5. For combination foods such as sandwiches, casseroles, and soups indicate the ingredients contained in the food. For example, a turkey sandwich may be described as 2 slices of whole wheat bread, 1 oz of smoked turkey, 1 slice of tomato, 2 leaves of iceberg lettuce, 1 T mayonnaise.
6. Indicate where, when, and with whom the meal or snack was eaten. Describe any feelings at the time of consumption whenever possible (e.g. worried, content, bored, lonely, stressed, etc.). This will help identify possible negative behavior as it relates to food consumption.
7. Indicate any physiological experiences such as level of hunger, thirst, or having a particular craving.

*Carry the following recording charts and write down foods as they are consumed. You may elect to photocopy the forms for ease of use. A sample record has been included to assist you with proper recording.

Sample Food Log

Amount (Serving Size)	Food Description (Cooking Method, Brand Name)	Location (Place, People, Social Environment)	Feeling (Hunger, Anger, Joy)	Time of Day
1 Cup	Kellogg's Corn Flakes	Home Breakfast table	Hungry	8 am
1/2 Cup	Low Fat milk 2%	Home Breakfast table	Hungry	8 am
1 Cup	Decaf Coffee	Home Breakfast table	Hungry	8 am
1	Banana	Home Breakfast table	Hungry	8 am

Food Log

Amount (Serving Size)	Food Description (Cooking Method, Brand Name)	Location (Place, People, Social Environment)	Feeling (Hunger, Anger, Joy)	Time of Day

Step 4   Perform a nutritional assessment and comparison using the DRI-RDA for Nutrients and Daily Caloric Need computation. You may utilize the Trainer Tools section of the NCSF website to assist you with your analysis. Go to www.ncsf.org and click on "Trainer Tools." Choose "Interactive Healthy Eating Index" and follow the directions to begin your analysis. If you are not an NCSF member go to **www.mypyramidtracker.gov** and click on "Assess Your Food Intake." Follow the detailed instructions to enter your data.

Analysis of food intake data following the 24-hour dietary log provides the health professional with the ability to make formal recommendations regarding the nutrient intake of their clients. The health professional should compare collected data against the recommended RDA intakes. In addition, if more than one day is used, the average daily caloric intake can be assessed for compliance with recommendations related to daily intake goals. Adjustments can then be made to the caloric intake to ensure adequate nutrients are consumed when caloric modifications are made. In this particular lab, the comparisons will be made to the USRDA using either food tables or a computerized diet-analysis program. The following list identifies the specific nutrient concerns health fitness professionals must recognize to make the proper recommendations.

- Total calories
- Average daily caloric intake
- Percentage of diet from carbohydrates
- Percentage of diet from protein
- Percentage of diet from fat
- Percentage of diet from simple sugar
- Percentage of diet from saturated fat

- Grams of fiber in diet
- Milligrams of Cholesterol
- Milligrams of Sodium
- Antioxidant consumption
- Appropriate vitamin intake
- Appropriate mineral intake
- Proper hydration status

Individuals with anthropometric measures that suggest an over-consumption of calories, but whose dietary recall indicates perfect food consumption habits should raise suspicion about the actual dietary intakes. Asking questions related to the data may provide evidence of recording errors or other unintentional mistakes. Clients suspected of under reporting, deliberately falsifying information, or altering customary intakes for the diet record should be asked directly if any possible errors may have occurred. Individuals unwilling to complete the dietary recall correctly should not participate in the assessment because it will serve little purpose for the fitness professional.

Activity 3.4 Dietary Analysis

Activity Description

On the following form record the subject's personal data and anthropometric measures. Then, refer to the subject's dietary log data to complete the analysis chart on the following page. Be sure to record all values in the appropriate spaces. Upon completion, review the chart with the subject and identify any areas of deficiency. Remember, when using a 3-day log you should take the average of the three days for each class of nutrient ingested.

Subject Data

Name _____   Gender _____

Date _____

Age _____   Weight _____lb   Weight _____kg

                  Height _____in   Height _____cm

Percentage of Body Fat _____%

Total Daily Caloric Intake _____ calories

Procedure

Step 1   Current Intake – Record subject's average intake using the correct unit of measure
Step 2   RDA – Record the RDA for each specific nutrient
Step 3   Food Sources – Identify two food sources that are high in the respective nutrient

Nutrient	Current Intake	DRI	Food Sources	Nutrient	Current Intake	DRI	Food Sources
Carbohydrates				Simple Sugars			
Fats				Saturated Fats			
Protein				Cholesterol			
Water (oz)				Fiber			
Vitamin A (μg R.E.)				Calcium (mg)			
Vitamin E (μg)[e]				Phosphorus (mg)			
Vitamin K (μg)				Magnesium (mg)			
Vitamin C (μg)				Iron (mg)			
Thiamin (mg)				Zinc (mg)			
Riboflavin (mg)				Iodine (μg)			
Niacin (mg N.E.)[f]				Selenium (μg)			
Vitamin B$_6$ (mg)				Choline (mg)			
Folate (μg)				Flouride (mg)			
Vitamin B$_{12}$ (μg)				Molybdenum (μg)			
Biotin				Chromium (μg)			
Alcoholic Beverages (oz)				Sodium (mg)			

Step 4   The information on the following chart is based upon an individual calculated need. You should have already calculated a daily caloric need and energy intakes based on activity levels during the performance of the prior activity sections (activity 3.2). Enter the data in the space labeled "Calculated Need."

Step 5   Enter the reported intakes from the dietary log.

Energy Nutrients	Reported Intake	Calculated Need	+ or – (amount)
Total Calories			
Calories From Fat			
Calories From CHO			
Calories From Protein			

Step 6   Determine if adjustments are required for the energy nutrients.

Activity 3.5 Assessing Hydration Status

Activity Description

Water comprises 60%-70% of bodyweight. It accounts for three quarters of the weight of muscle and constitutes more than half of the weight of adipose tissue. Variations in total body fluid occur among individuals with different tissue compositions. Water plays a role in most actions that occur within the body. It serves as a transport and reactive medium, aids in the diffusion of gases, facilitates digestive mobility, mixes with other constituents to lubricate and reduce frictional coefficients within the body, and is the primary factor in the regulation of heat. The body relies on adequate amounts of water to serve the many interactive roles to maintain proper homeostasis. If water consumption does not meet requirements, the body fails to function properly.

A relationship exists between water and minerals within the body, which make their daily consumption very important. Minerals need water to form electrolytes in the body. In turn, water needs minerals to maintain fluid balance inside and outside of the cell membrane. When water dissolves minerals they become ions, or electrolytes. The term electrolyte is given to these ions because they have an electrical charge and conduct electricity. When these electrical conductors are maintained in correct concentration within the cell and outside of the cell, water balance should be maintained. The loss of water and electrolytes is elevated during exercise. When high intensity exercise is performed or exercise is performed in heated conditions the loss is further increased. To maintain adequate hydration status exercisers and athletes should track their water intake and loss during exercise.

Procedures

The act of calculating fluid loss for the maintenance of physiological homeostasis can be accomplished relatively easily. Monitoring bodyweight before and after an exercise bout allows the fitness professional to make more accurate recommendations for fluid replenishment.

The following section will require you to chart fluid loss rates in response to physical activity. Read through the following steps and perform all designated procedures.

Step 1   Using an accurate scale, weigh yourself, or a subject, just prior to exercise and record the weight in kilograms.

Pre-exercise body weight in pounds ÷ 2.2 = _____ kg

Step 2   Perform moderate to vigorous exercise for a period of thirty minutes or more. Be sure to pre-measure and record any fluids ingested during the activity. Do not go to the bathroom between the period of pre-exercise weigh-in and post-exercise weigh-in because it will distort fluid volume changes.

Record exercise duration _____ minutes

Record fluid intake _____ ounces

Step 3   Once the training has been completed, wait 5 minutes for post-exercise temperature regulation to occur and re-weigh test subject. Record the weight in kilograms.

Post-exercise bodyweight in pounds ÷ 2.2 = _____ kg

Step 4   Complete the chart to determine the actual sweat rate for the exercise duration (Step 5).

Name	Date	BW Pre-Exercise	BW Post Exercise	Pre- Post BW Diff	Fluid Consumed	Sweat Loss	Exercise Duration	Sweat Rate
Sample	8/20	100 kg	99 kg	1000 g	500 ml (17 oz)	1500 Ml	60 min	25 ml/min

Modified from GSSI, 9:(4 Suppl 63),1996

Step 5   Calculate sweat loss.

(Pre BW - Post BW) + Fluid Consumed = Sweat Loss

_____ - _____ + _____ = _____ ml Sweat loss

Step 6   Calculate sweat rate.

Sweat Loss _____ ml ÷ Exercise Duration _____ min. = Sweat Rate (ml • min^{-1})

Step 7   Multiply the Sweat Rate (ml/min) x 60 minutes to calculate milliliters per hour

Sweat Rate x 60 minutes = _____ ml • hr^{-1}

Step 8   Using the chart below, determine the fluid replenishment schedule for the test subject.

Sweat Rate ml • hr^{-1}	Fluid Intake		Rehydration Intervals
	ml	oz	
500	125	4.0	15
750	190	6.5	15
1000	250	8.5	15
1500	250	8.5	10
2000	330	11.0	10
2500	415	14.0	10
3000	500	17.0	10

Recommended fluid intake during exercise: _____ ml every _____ minutes

Lab Three Submission Form – Nutritional Assessment

1. How many calories are in a food containing 20 grams of fat, 16 grams of protein, and 30 grams of carbohydrate?

_____ Total Calories

2. What percentage of total calories comes from fat sources in the above food?

_____%

3. What fuel serves as the primary source for physical activity and represents the largest portion of the normal diet?

_____

4. Explain why endurance athletes require more protein than individuals who are physically active.

_____

_____

_____

5. What is the recommended intake for fat for physically active persons? _____%

6. Using the following information, calculate the recommended carbohydrate and protein consumption, in grams, for a male football player weighing 220 lbs (Assume 1.6 g/kg of bodyweight for protein).

Calculated Daily Caloric Intake Requirement	4987 kcal
Recommended CHO Intake	60%
Recommended carbohydrate grams	_____ grams
Recommended carbohydrate calories	_____ Kcals
Recommended protein grams	_____ grams
Recommended protein calories	_____ Kcals

7. Case study: Your new client has the following physical characteristics:

Gender	Female
Height	5' 2"
Weight	165 lbs
BF %	32
Age	45
Activity	Sedentary – no reported physical activity
Goal	Weight loss

Lab Three Submission Form – Nutritional Assessment

After analyzing the 24 hour recall for the above client, you find that they have consumed 400 grams of carbohydrates, 100 grams of protein, and 50 grams of fat.

A. How many calories did they consume?   _____

B. What percentage of calories came from fat?   _____

C. What percentage of calories came from carbohydrates?   _____

D. What percentage of calories came from protein?   _____

8. List three common user errors when implementing food logs?

1. _____

2. _____

3. _____

9. Attach a copy of the food log used in activity 3.3 and the dietary analysis from activity 3.4.

10. What is the relationship between minerals and water?

_____

_____

_____

Lab Four
Body Composition and Weight Management

Lab Four corresponds to the following textbook readings:

Body Composition	Chapter 10
Weight Management	Chapter 11

Lab Description

Body composition is a term that refers to the constitutional make-up of the human body. It quantifies the tissue components by compartments. When the term is used as a health related component of fitness, it categorizes tissue into two primary compartments: fat mass and fat-free mass. Fat mass (FM), as the name implies, encompasses all the fat found in the body including fat stored subcutaneously, surrounding vital organs, and embedded in the muscle. Fat-free mass (FFM) is then defined as anything that is not fat (i.e. muscle, bone, connective tissue, etc.). Lean mass is often used interchangeably with fat-free mass. This is mildly erroneous, as lean mass includes as much as 3% of essential fat stores. Essential fats are lipids stored in the body's organs, muscle, bone marrow, and tissues of the nervous system. They are necessary for normal physiological function. Collectively with storage fat, they make up the fat mass of the body.

Researchers have developed numerous methods to estimate a person's body fat using direct and indirect assessments. Numerous types of body composition assessment protocols exist and each offers different positive and negative aspects associated with their employment as evaluative instruments. The most common body composition assessment methods are field tests based on anthropometric measurements such as skinfold or circumference measurements. Additionally, recent technology based assessments using bioelectrical impedance analysis (BIA) and near-infrared interactance (NIR) have become popular in the fitness settings. Personal trainers must identify the differences in predictive value and understand the variables that affect the true measurement of body fat, as accuracy varies between methods.

Field assessments of body composition estimate fat mass based on predictive equations and comparative norms. Field tests have obvious benefits for the personal trainer as most methods are affordable, can be performed in numerous environments, require limited technical training compared to laboratory methods, and have reasonable prediction accuracy. The final choice for selection of the body composition method will be based upon tester proficiency, availability of equipment, and relative need for accuracy.

Explored Procedures

- Stature/Weight Index (BMI)
- 2-3 Girth estimation of body fat
- Skinfold estimation of body fat
- Calculation of lean body mass
- Calculation of target weight
- Calculation of resting metabolic rate

Lab Objectives

- Understand and apply the information related to anthropometric measurements and disease risk stratification
- Accurately assess body composition using the procedures outlined in this lab
- Calculate fat-free mass based on measured body composition
- Analyze results and be able to make recommendations based on current body fat percentages
- Determine target body weight
- Calculate resting metabolic rate and predicted daily need
- Be able to apply the information to program prescription and goal setting

Activity 4.1 Body Mass Index (BMI)

Activity Description

Stature/Weight Indices compare the height of an individual to their weight and formulate conclusions based upon this relationship. Values are often compared to healthy weight ranges for specific populations based on all-cause morbidity and risks associated with deviations from healthy weight ranges. The predictions are based upon population norms and morbidity rates using height and weight ratios. They do not directly measure the amount of fat or lean mass on the body. The drawbacks to this are obvious. A person may have large amounts of lean mass and a relatively low quantity of body fat causing their weight to be dramatically higher than someone who has greater fat mass and less muscle. This would predict them as having an unhealthy weight and classify them in a higher risk category even though they may actually be very healthy.

Body Mass Index (BMI) is the most common stature/weight index used to categorize people for risk of disease based on anthropometrics. The effectiveness of the BMI formula lies in its curvilinear relationship to the all-cause mortality ratio. The original formula uses a subject's mass (kg) divided by stature, height squared (m^2). A newer formula using English measurement units may be found to be easier for some people. Interpreting the BMI score as a measurement of body fat provides limited value, as proportional composition variables are not directly assessed. The norms for the BMI may imply that the higher the BMI of an individual, the greater the percentage of fat, but as stated earlier this may not always be the case, particularly for subjects with higher amounts of muscle mass. BMI's primary role is to serve as a clinical assessment tool to measure the appropriateness of a person's weight in relation to height. The lowest risk for disease is found within the BMI range of 20 to 25, with values exceeding 40 considered the highest risk. It has been suggested that the most desirable range is between 21.9 and 22.4 for males and between 21.3 and 22.1 for females. When BMI values surpass 27.8 for males and 27.3 for females the risk of hypertension, diabetes, and coronary artery disease increases. A person is considered overweight when their BMI is between 25 and 30 and obese when the value is greater than 30.

Procedures

Complete the following activity using the procedures detailed below. You may use either the English or Metric formulas. Once a BMI value has been calculated for your test subject, reference the score using the tables in Chapter 10 to evaluate results.

Step 1   Measure and record subject's weight:

_____ lbs.

_____ kg

Step 2   Measure and record subject's height:

_____ inches

_____ meters

Conversions
1 in = .0254 meters
1 kg = 2.2 lbs.

Sample

5' 10" 150 lb female

$150 \div 2.2 = 68$ kg

70 inches x .0254 = 1.778 m

Perform your conversion for the Metric formula below:

_____ lbs ÷ 2.2 = _____ kg

_____ inches x .0254 = _____ m

Step 3   Calculate your subject's BMI using one of the following formulas.

English Formula: BMI = {Weight (lbs) ÷ Height (inches)^2} x 703

Metric Formula: BMI = Weight (kg) ÷ Height (meters)^2

Example One (English)

5"10 in. 150 lbs. female

BMI = {150 lbs ÷ (70 inches)^2} x 703

BMI = (150 ÷ 4900) x 703

BMI = 0.0306 x 703

BMI = 21.5

Example Two (Metric)

5"10 in. 150 lbs. female

1.778 m 68 kg female

BMI = 68 ÷ (1.788)^2

BMI = 68 ÷ 3.196

BMI = 21.3

Perform your calculation below by selecting one of the two calculation methods:

BMI = { _____ lbs. ÷ (_____ inches)^2 }x 703   **Or**   BMI = _____ kg ÷ (_____ m)^2

BMI = (_____ lbs. ÷ _____) x 703   BMI = _____ kg ÷ _____

BMI = _____   BMI = _____

Step 4   Reference the BMI tables on page 174 of the course textbook to interpret your results.

Activity 4.2 2-3 Girth Estimation of Body Fat

Activity Description

Circumference estimation of body composition employs measurements of select locations to predict body fat. The methods are easy to perform and require minimal equipment. The assessment device is often no more than a common linen or plastic measuring tape. Often referred to as "girth measurements," they simply require the circumference measurement of designated sites of the body. The measured values are then charted, graphed, or equated based on the particular protocol being used. Depending upon the estimation model, girth measurements can predict body composition and help determine regional fat storage. The estimations are based on the positive linear relationship between the circumference values of particular anatomical areas and the amount of body fat a person carries.

Girth measurements are very practical assessment methods for fitness professionals and are considered psychologically benign for most clients. When performed correctly with the appropriate prediction equation, circumference estimations of body fat can have a *SEE* of as little as ± 2.5% - 4%. They also provide useful information about fat distribution patterns as well as body fat changes during weight loss. Clients can see and understand the quantifiable differences found between measurements, which often serve as motivation even when bodyweight remains unchanged. Additionally, the methods are far more useful for measuring and predicting the body fat of obese individuals, as skinfold and other methods lose predictive value with higher levels of adipose tissue.

The 2-3 Girth estimation of body fat is based on information gathered by the Naval Health Research Center (NHRC) and was developed from the data collected on large samples of Navy men and women. The model has been found to have high correlations ($r = 0.85$ and 0.90) and reasonable standard errors ($SEE = 3.7\%$ and 2.7%) when compared to hydrostatic weighing. The 2-3 Girth estimation is based on the linear relationship between circumference measurements and body fat. In the 2-3 Girth method, the neck represents the reference value for lean body mass in both male and female models, whereas the abdominal and hip girths represent the fat factor for the prediction.

Procedures

Follow the directions below to compute the 2-3 Girth estimation of body fat using a volunteer subject.

Step 1   *Anthropometric data collection.* Measure the appropriate anatomical locations of the subject and record the value in the space provided (Reference p294 in Chapter 14 of your textbook for a detailed overview).

All circumference measurements should be taken over the subject's skin where applicable. Tight fitting clothing should be worn when skin contact is not appropriate.

Men

- Abdominal measurement - measure the circumference of the abdomen by aligning the tape so that it passes over the navel.
- Neck - measure the circumference of the neck just inferior to the larynx (Adam's apple).
- Record your results.

Abdominal circumference	_____ in.
Neck circumference	_____ in.
Height	_____ in.

Women

- Upper abdominal measurement - measure the circumference of the upper abdomen by aligning the tape so that it is between the distal aspect of the rib cage and the navel.
- Hip - measure the circumference of the hip in the center of the gluteals at the level of the greater Trochanter, or curvilinear apex, of the hip (widest points).
- Neck - measure the circumference of the neck just inferior to the larynx.
- Record your results.

Upper abdominal circumference	_____ in.
Hip circumference	_____ in.
Neck circumference	_____ in.
Height	_____ in.

Step 2   *Calculate subject's derived circumference value.* The 2-3 Girth model utilizes a derived circumference value to ascertain the subject's estimated body fat. From the data collected in Step 1, find the subject's derived circumference value by utilizing the following gender specific equation.

Men: Abdominal – Neck = Circumference value

_____ – _____ = _____

Women: Upper abdominal + Hip – Neck = Circumference value

_____ + _____ – _____ = _____

Step 3   *Find subject's estimated 2-3 Girth percent body fat.* The charts in Chapter 14 contain the estimated body fat percentages according to the 2-3 Girth model. To find your subject's estimated body fat you must first refer to the correct gender table (Table A for men and Table B for women). You must then match the subject's calculated circumference value from Step 2 with the subject's height in inches. The derived circumference values are located in the left hand column and the height values are located across the top of the table.

Step 4   *Record data.* Record the subject's estimated 2-3 Girth percent body fat value.

_____ Body fat percentage

Step 5   *Interpret the data.* Compare the subject's predicted body fat measurement with the body fat percentage chart on p182 in Chapter 10.

Activity 4.3 Skinfold Estimation of Body Fat

Activity Description

One of the most popular methods of assessing body fat employs the use of calipers to measure the thickness of subcutaneous adipose tissue in various locations of the body. Subcutaneous fat is stored between the muscle and dermal layer of skin. It represents about 50%-70% of total body fat stored in the body. The remaining fat surrounds various vital organs, is embedded within the tissues in and around muscle, and circulates in the blood stream. Through the use of regression equations, it is possible to predict the amount of fat mass a person has by measuring the thickness of skinfolds at specific sites.

There are several protocols to choose from when assessing an individual's body composition with calipers. The most common protocols use 2, 3, or 7 sites for predictive value. Three site analysis has been shown to have a better predictive value than two sites, and using more than three sites has not conclusively shown to increase the accuracy of the assessment. Skinfold equations are typically within 4% of the value measured using underwater weighing.

Assessing body composition by means of skinfold analysis requires a high degree of technical expertise and the technique of measuring skinfolds requires considerable practice; the technician must familiarize him or herself with the feel of the subcutaneous fold. This expertise is developed through continual practice on different subjects, as individual differences in the consistency of fat mass exist. Factors to consider include skinfold compressibility, skin tightness, edema, and variability in fat distribution. This supports the need for repeated practice before a technician becomes proficient at the technique and obviously suggests that the tester's expertise and adherence to the administration protocol affects the *SEE* of this methodology.

Calibration and pincher selection will also affect the measurement. Pincher tension should be set at a constant 10 g · mm^{-2}. Calipers that use manually controlled pincher tension should be avoided for accurate assessment, as the actual tension cannot be reliably controlled. Additionally, the location of the fold measurement and speed of the reading can also affect accuracy. The fold should be measured in accordance with the description that follows to increase the accuracy of the measurement. A rapid reading is also important as fat is compressible and will "seep out" under the tension of the pinchers, therefore reducing the measure and subsequent prediction. Individuals that have excessive fat mass should be measured with girth measurements or similar replacement methods.

This lab will examine a 3-site measurement procedure formulated by Jackson and Pollock. The model measures the thickness of the subcutaneous fat in the chest, abdomen, and thigh of males and triceps, suprailiac, and thigh of females. It is critical that the site of the skinfold measurement be accurately determined and marked before the assessment begins. This will increase the accuracy of the measurement. The site for measurement should be located and then marked with an erasable marker. This will help ensure that the calipers are placed precisely in the correct position each time the skinfold is measured. The exact location for the pinch and placement of the caliper will be explained in greater detail in the procedures section.

Procedures

Follow the description below to calculate the percent body fat for a sample subject using the 3-site skinfold method. Answer the corresponding activity questions at the end of the section.

Step 1   *Locate the correct gender-specific anatomical location(s).* The following chart and illustrations on p288-290 in Chapter 14 provide a detailed description of the 3-site Jackson and Pollock model. Refer to these when locating the correct gender specific skinfold locations. Once the site has been identified, mark the site with an erasable marker so that you can return to the exact location for subsequent measurements. This will also allow you to become more proficient at site identification and increase test reliability. **Note**: You may need to wipe the area dry of oils, sweat, or lotions before marking the site.

Jackson and Pollock Gender-Specific Skinfold Sites

- Men – Chest, Abdominal, Thigh
- Women – Tricep, Suprailiac, Thigh

Site Locations	Fold Orientation	Fold Description
Abdomen	Vertical	Taken 2 cm (approximately 1 in.) to the right of the umbilicus.
Chest (*Males only*)	Diagonal	The site is one half the distance between the anterior axillary line and the nipple.
Thigh	Vertical	On the front of the thigh, midway between the hip (inguinal crease) and the superior aspect of the patella (kneecap).
Tricep	Vertical	Located halfway between the acromion process (shoulder) and the inferior part of the elbow on the rear midline of the upper arm.
Suprailiac	Diagonal	Taken with the natural angle of the iliac crest at the anterior axillary line immediately superior to the iliac crest.

Step 2   *Hand placement.* Place the caliper in the right hand with the index finger in a position to open the caliper. Slightly pronate the right hand so that the caliper can be easily read from above. Pronate the left hand to a point at which the thumb of the left hand is pointing downward. A simplified description is to have the tester place both arms out in front of him/her and rotate both arms inward so that both thumbs are pointing downward, with the caliper in the right hand. With the thumb and forefinger facing downward, place the thumb and finger perpendicular to the marked site of the skinfold.

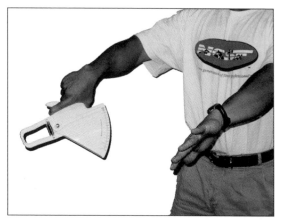

Step 3   *Pinching of skinfold.* Using a pinch width of approximately two inches wide, firmly pinch the skinfold between the thumb and first two fingers, lifting the subcutaneous fat and skin from the underlying muscle tissue.

Step 4   *Placement of calipers.* Once the tester has successfully separated the subcutaneous fat and skin from the underlying muscle belly, the calipers should be placed on the fold. The pinchers of the caliper should be placed across the long axis of the skinfold at the designated site. Using a 1 cm separation between the technician's fingers and the calipers should prevent the skinfold dimension from being affected by the pressure from the tester's fingers. The depth of caliper placement is about half the distance between the base of the normal skin perimeter and the top of the skinfold. Place the jaws of the calipers perpendicular to the skinfold site approximately 1 cm below the fingers. This will allow the caliper reading to be done approximately halfway between the bottom and top of the fold.

Step 5   *Reading of calipers.* Calipers have a compression tension of $10 \text{ g} \cdot \text{mm}^2$. In order to get an accurate reading and prevent compression of the fat by the caliper, the tester must read the caliper to the closest half millimeter within 2 seconds of applying the caliper jaws to the fold. Measure each site and record the assessment values on the Data Recording Sheet. The measurements should be repeated two times allowing at least 15 seconds between subsequent measurements. If the measurements differ by more than 2 millimeters, a third measurement should be taken and an average of the three measurements used. In non-obese individuals, the skinfolds should not differ by more than two millimeters. The median values of the three trials are used for evaluation and prediction.

Step 6   *Record results.* Record the individual site measurements on the provided data recording form. The measurements will be used to compare future assessment results.

3-Site Skinfold Body Composition Estimation Data Recording Form

Men: Trial 1   Chest _____   Abdominal _____   Thigh _____

Trial 2   Chest _____   Abdominal _____   Thigh _____

Trial 3   Chest _____   Abdominal _____   Thigh _____

Average _____   Average _____   Average _____

Sum of the Three Averages _____

Women: Trial 1   Tricep _____   Suprailium _____   Thigh _____

Trial 2   Tricep _____   Suprailium _____   Thigh _____

Trial 3   Tricep _____   Suprailium _____   Thigh _____

Average _____   Average _____   Average _____

Sum of the three averages _____

Step 7   *Computation of results.* Once the data has been recorded on the provided Data Recording Sheet, the tester should add the three skinfolds together to obtain the sum of skinfolds in millimeters. The sum of the skinfolds is then charted or used in a body density equation to determine the estimated body fat of the individual. The charts on p291-292 in Chapter 14 contain the estimated age-adjusted body composition computed by the Siri Equation. Find your subject's estimated body fat by referencing the gender-specific table; by matching the sum of the skinfolds in the left hand column with the subject's age on the top row.

Estimated Body Fat _____ %

Step 8   *Interpretation of results.* After the subject has been classified by estimated value, the results can be used to establish goals and develop weight management strategies. Listed below are general classifications for body fat.

Percent Fat in Men and Women

Risk Category	Men (% Body Fat)	Women (% Body Fat)
Essential	3-5	11-14.9
Lean	6-10.9	15-18.9
Fitness	11-15.9	19-22.9
Healthy	16-19.9	23-26.9
Moderate Risk	20-24.9	27-31.9
High Risk	>25	>32

Activity 4.4 Calculating Lean Mass & Target Body Weight

Activity Description

Differentiating the tissue compartments by mass is useful in determining the necessary changes for optimal health and goal setting for weight loss or gain. Using the percentage of body fat determined via body composition analysis personal trainers can identify the relative quantity of lean and fat mass on the body. These values can then be used to calculate target weight for appropriate adjustments in body composition.

Procedures

Following the instructions below, enter the appropriate data to calculate lean mass and target body weight. Use the examples provided for guidance.

Calculating Lean Mass

Bodyweight x Body fat percentage = Fat mass

Bodyweight – Fat mass = Lean mass

Example

200 lb. male 20% body fat

200 lbs. x 0.20 = 40 lbs.

Fat mass = 40 lbs.

200 lbs – 40 lbs. = 160 lbs.

Lean mass = 160 lbs.

Step 1   Enter estimated body fat _____ %

Enter bodyweight _____ lbs.

Step 2   Enter the values from Step 1 into the formula.

Estimated body fat (_____ % ÷ 100) x bodyweight _____ lbs. = _____ Fat mass

Step 3   Calculate lean mass by subtracting the fat mass, in pounds, from the total body weight.

Bodyweight _____ lbs. – Fat mass _____ lbs. = Lean mass _____ lbs.

Calculating Target Body Weight

Using the formula provided, calculate the Target Body Weight for a volunteer subject or the sample subject below. The formula will identify the weight of the individual at the selected body fat percentage assuming the weight lost is fat mass and not lean mass.

Lean Mass ÷ {1 - (desired body fat percent ÷ 100)} = Target Body Weight

Example

200 lb man 20% body fat

Lean Mass 160 lbs.

New desired body fat 18%

160 lbs. ÷ {1-(18% ÷ 100)} = Target Body Weight

160 lbs. ÷ {1- (.18)} = Target Body Weight

160 lbs. ÷ (.82) = 195 lbs.

200 lbs. − 195 lbs. = 5 lbs. weight loss

Procedures

Using the sample subject below or a volunteer subject, calculate the desired body weight for a 3% reduction in body fat.

Sample Subject: Jennifer is 32 years old and weighs 145 lbs. Her current body composition is 28%. Her short-term goal is 25%.

Step 1   Calculate Fat Mass using the formula below.

Enter Current Body Weight   _____ lbs.

Enter Current Body Fat   _____ %

Estimated body fat (_____% ÷ 100) x Body weight _____ lbs. = _____ Fat mass

Step 2   Calculate lean mass by subtracting the fat mass in pounds from the total body weight.

Body weight _____ lbs. – Fat mass _____ lbs. = Lean mass _____ lbs.

Enter Lean Mass _____ lbs.

Step 3   Select a new Desired Body Fat   _____ %

Step 4   Enter the values from Step 1 and Step 2 into the formula below to calculate the Target Body Weight. Hint: Do not convert the body fat percentage into a decimal before inserting the value.

Lean Mass _____ lbs. ÷ {1- (desired body fat percent _____ ÷ 100)} = Target Body Weight

Lean Mass _____ lbs. ÷ {1- (_____)} = Target Body Weight

Lean Mass _____ lbs. ÷ _____ = _____ Target Body Weight

Step 5   Subtract the Target Body Weight from the initial body weight to identify the weight loss goals.

Current body weight _____ – Target Body Weight _____ = Weight loss goal _____ lbs.

Once the initial short-term goal has been attained, the personal trainer must then re-compute the target body weight based on new desired body fat goals.

Step 6   In the chart below, calculate the desired weight for the subject as they lose body fat. Bodyweight should reflect a specific duration of time, reasonable fat loss goals, and account for the maintenance of lean mass. **Note**: Lean mass should not change during the calculation of predicted weight loss and body fat goals.

Example

Starting Value 08/03/2008	Goal #1 09/07/2008	Goal #2 10/12/2008	Goal #3 11/15/2008
22%	20%	18%	16%
190 lb	185.25 lb	180.7 lb	176.4 lb

Desired Body Weight

Starting Value Dates	Goal #1	Goal #2	Goal #3
_____%	_____%	_____%	_____%
_____lb	_____lb	_____lb	_____lb

Activity 4.5 Individual Metabolic Needs Assessment

Activity Description

Metabolic assessment describes a variety of methods used to determine relevant information related to a subject's metabolic fitness and energy requirement. Health is dependent upon maintaining the sometimes delicate balance between suitable body fuel to support energy needs and satisfying nutritional requirements to sustain proper biological function without adding adipose tissue. Utilizing the proper assessment tools enable the personal trainer to identify possible areas that need to be addressed to help balance caloric requirements for varying clients' needs.

Metabolic Rate is defined as the rate at which we expend energy (calories) to facilitate the demands of the body's tissue. Resting Metabolic Rate (RMR) can be defined as the amount of energy (calories) needed to sustain the bodily functions under normal resting conditions. Each action that occurs within the body, whether physiological or biochemical, requires energy to support its activity. This energy generates heat, which can be measured using Direct Calorimetry in a research laboratory. Researchers use this method to determine the specific energy costs of physiological activities. This form of assessment is very accurate, but comes with a considerable monetary cost and large scale delivery limitations. A less expensive version of calorimetry used to measure caloric expenditure is known as Spirometry or Indirect Calorimetry. This method analyzes oxygen utilization rather than heat production as the measurable criteria. Spirometry estimates the heat using the quantity of oxygen inhaled and carbon dioxide exhaled into a special breathing device. The caloric expenditure can be calculated using the Respiratory Exchange Ratio (R) from the caloric equivalent of oxygen utilized.

Although these methods are very accurate and provide valuable data for the researchers in clinical lab settings, they have little relevance in the majority of personal training environments. Fortunately, there have been several additional methods developed to estimate metabolic rate. Using the scientific information gathered from researchers, we can now estimate metabolic rates through the use of predictive formulas.

Due to the fact that RMR comprises approximately 60% to 70% of a person's daily caloric need, it is important for persons engaging in weight loss, weight maintenance, or weight gain programs to know the approximate caloric intake needed for goal attainment. Through the estimation of RMR using the Harris-Benedict Formula or the Lean Mass Formula, a personal trainer can estimate the amount of calories a person needs to sustain current body weight in a normal resting condition. The personal trainer can then assess the client's general activity level and make adjustments using the corresponding activity multiplier to calculate the Daily Caloric Need. This step is very important, as people do not regularly lay in bed all day.

Procedures

Using yourself or lab partner as a subject, follow the steps below to calculate RMR using the RMR Prediction Equation and the estimation of Daily Caloric Need. A 50-year-old, 215 pound, 6 feet tall, male subject is used as an example to assist you in the steps.

Harris-Benedict Equation

- Males: $66 + (5 \times ht) + (13.8 \times wt) - (6.8 \times age)$

- Females: $655 + (1.8 \times ht) + (9.6 \times wt) - (4.7 \times age)$

   - RMR expressed in kilocalories per day
   - HT (Height) expressed in centimeters
   - WT (Weight) expressed in kilograms
   - Age expressed in years

Example Conversions

215 pound male subject

$215 \div 2.2$ lb/kg $= 97.7$ kg

Sample 6 foot tall subject

6 ft x 12 inches/ft = 72 inches

72 inches x 2.54 cm/in = 182.9 cm

Sample subject's RMR calculation

RMR $= 66 + (5 \times ht) + (13.8 \times wt) - (6.8 \times age)$

RMR $= 66 + (5 \times 182.9) + (13.8 \times 97.7) - (6.8 \times 50)$

RMR $= 1988$ kcal per day

Step 1   Convert subject's body weight from pounds to kilograms

Test Subject's weight _____ lbs.

_____ lbs. $\div 2.2$ lb/kg $=$ _____ kg

Step 2   Convert height in inches to centimeters

Test Subject's height _____ inches

_____ inches x 2.54 cm/in = _____ cm

Step 3   Calculate RMR in the spaces provided below by using your numbers from Steps 1 and 2 above. Be sure to use the correct gender formula.

RMR Males

RMR = 66 + (5 x ht) + (13.8 x wt) – (6.8 x age)

RMR = 66 + (5 x _____ cm) + (13.8 x _____ kg) – (6.8 x _____ years)

RMR = 66 + (_____) + (_____) – (_____)

RMR = _____ kcals

RMR Females

RMR = 655 + (1.8 x ht) + (9.6 x wt) – (4.7 x age)

RMR = 655 + (1.8 x _____ cm) + (9.6 x _____ kg) – (4.7 x _____ years)

RMR = 655 + (_____) + (_____) – (_____)

RMR = _____ kcals

Estimated RMR for your test subject: _____ (kcal)

Lean Mass Estimation of RMR

The amount of lean mass a person carries influences RMR. It is widely accepted that muscle is more metabolically active than fat, even during resting conditions. This suggests that if two individuals weigh the same, the person with the higher amount of fat-free mass (FFM), or greater lean body weight (LBW), should have a higher RMR than the person with a higher amount of fat mass (FM). This further supports the need for a resistance training component in a fitness program aimed at weight loss.

Following the steps below, calculate the RMR value for your test subject. Use their body fat results from Lab 4.2 or 4.3 to calculate RMR using the lean mass equation.

Step 1   Determine lean mass value of subject using body composition analysis

Test Subject's weight in pounds _____

Test Subject's body fat percentage _____

Percent body fat x _____ weight in pounds = _____ Fat mass

Weight in pounds – _____ Fat mass = _____ Fat-free mass

Step 2   Determine Fat-free mass in kilograms

Fat-free mass in lbs._____ ÷ 2.2 = _____ Fat-free mass in kilograms

Step 3   Calculate RMR from Fat-free mass using the following formula

RMR (kcal/day) = 370 + (21.6 x fat-free mass in kg)

RMR (kcal/day) = 370 + (21.6 x _____ kg)

RMR (kcal/day) = 370 + (_____)

RMR = _____

Step 4   Compare Lean Mass RMR value to the Harris-Benedict RMR Predication Equation value.

Predicted RMR _____

Activity 4.6 Daily Caloric Need

Activity Description

Once RMR is known, the Daily Caloric Need can be determined to identify a person's predicted caloric requirements. RMR only represents the amount of calories a person expends at rest and it is a reasonable assumption that a person will engage in some level of activity throughout the day. Whether the activities include normal daily living, i.e., walking, climbing stairs, shopping, working, or participation in a formal exercise routine, the amount of calories expended must be accounted for when calculating Daily Caloric Need. The Daily Caloric Need represents the amount of calories needed to sustain current body weight while factoring in average daily activities. It can be found by multiplying the RMR value from Step 3 of activity 4.5 by an Activity Factor coefficient. It is very important to choose an activity factor coefficient that best depicts the activity lifestyle of the client or an estimation error may occur. Most commonly, an overestimation of Daily Caloric Need occurs and leads to difficulty in weight loss goal attainment. The following tables will provide you with information pertaining to the classification of a subject and their daily caloric need based on reported activity. This information is important to the personal trainer, as it will aid in establishing the proper nutritional program to meet a client's needs and goals.

Procedures

Calculate your test subject's Daily Caloric Need by multiplying the RMR value from either the Harris-Benedict Equation or the Lean Mass Equation by the correct corresponding Activity Multiplier (see following table).

RMR (kcal) x Activity Multiplier (see below) = Daily Caloric Need

RMR _____ kcal x Activity multiplier _____ = Daily Caloric Need _____ calories

Level of Intensity	Type of Activity	Activity Factor (x RMR)	Energy Expenditure (kcal • kg • day)
Very light	Seated and standing activities, professional jobs, laboratory work, typing, sewing, ironing, and cooking	1.3 Women 1.4 Men	30 31
Light	Walking on a level surface at 2.5 to 3 mph, garage work, electrical trades, carpentry, restaurant trades, house cleaning, child care, golf, sailing, and table tennis	1.5 Women 1.6 Men	35 38
Moderate	Walking 3.5 to 4 mph, landscaping, carrying loads, cycling, skiing, tennis, and dancing	1.6 Women 1.7 Men	37 41
Heavy	Walking with load uphill, tree work, heavy manual digging, basketball, climbing, football, and soccer	1.9 Women 2.1 Men	44 50
Vigorous	Athletes training in professional or world-class events	2.2 Women 2.4 Men	51 58

It is quite obvious from the table that the more active an individual is, the higher the activity multiplier used will be. The activity multiplier can be adjusted to half-numbers (i.e. 1.45). You can use the table to "classify" your client's fitness level, but be aware that it is not uncommon for individuals to overestimate their activity level. For a personal trainer working with a client who has weight loss as the primary goal, it is recommended to use the lowest reasonable activity multiplier to best meet the caloric restriction requirements needed for weight loss.

Lab Four Submission Form – Body Composition and Weight Management

1. What are the two primary components of body composition?

    _____

    _____

2. Other than the fat stored subcutaneously, name two other places fat is found in the body.

    _____

    _____

3. In the spaces provided, calculate the BMI of a 6 feet tall, 200 lb man.

    BMI = {_____ lbs. ÷ (_____ inches $)^2$ } x 703

    BMI = {_____ lbs. ÷ _____ } x 703

    BMI = _____

4. According to the chart, what classification does this person fall under?

    _____

5. When BMI climbs above _____ kg/m^2, the risk of developing cardiovascular disease rises dramatically.

6. It is suggested that adults maintain a BMI below _____ kg/m^2.

7. The varying gender sites for the 2-3 Girth estimation were chosen based on:

    _____

    _____

8. Determine the body fat percentage of a 5'5" female with the following 2-3 Girth measurements.

    Circumference Values

    Neck   13"

    Upper abdominal   29"

    Hip circumference   37"

    Enter value here_____

Lab Four Submission Form – Body Composition and Weight Management

9. A 32-year-old female has the following caliper readings:

Triceps	38 mm
Suprailiac	25 mm
Thigh	50 mm

What is her estimated body fat according to the charts?

Enter answer here_____%

10. When is girth estimation of body composition a viable alternative to caliper estimation?

_____

_____

Lab Five
Health Appraisal & Screening Protocols

Lab Five corresponds to the following textbook readings:

Physical Fitness and Health	Chapter 12
Pre-exercise Screening and Test Considerations	Chapter 13

Lab Description

In the initial meeting with a prospective new client you are likely to discuss items such as previous workout experience, personal goals and expectations that they may have, what they are looking to gain from the personal trainer services, your fees and payment schedule, as well as a workout session schedule. Once the introductory consultation items have been discussed, and long before any exercise is performed, the trainer is expected to initiate non-exercise screening protocols. This entails the creation of the client profile which provides valuable knowledge about the client in accordance with the total fitness paradigm. This is extremely important as each client has specific characteristics and behaviors that set them apart from anyone else. This lends itself to the concept of individual profiling for successful health and fitness programming. Generic programming is not only inappropriate, but can have dramatic implications for risk management issues and your ability to meet specific individual requirements.

The screening process starts with the client completing an Informed Consent and proceeds to the completion of a Health Status Questionnaire and Behavior Form. Additionally, resting battery assessments will be evaluated in conjunction with findings on the forms to determine the appropriate steps to activity participation. These procedures are used in the initial development of the client's training profile. The information provided on these forms plays a vital role in addressing liability issues, training prescriptions, and the identification of negative behaviors and risk factors. The documents serve as part of the client's file and should be used for tracking and decision making throughout the course of the training program. All documents must be kept in a secure location and remain confidential as they contain personal and medical information. The following activities will direct you through the procedures to accurately identify risk factors and information relevant to program decisions.

Explored Procedures

- Identify risk factors for heart disease
- Implementation of the Informed Consent Form
- Implementation of the Health Status Questionnaire
- Implementation of Health Behavior Form

Lab Objectives

- Understand the role of an Informed Consent Form and the legal considerations for its use
- Understand the importance of confidentiality and file management
- Understand the role of a Health Status Questionnaire (HSQ)
- Be able to review the HSQ and identify possible contraindications to exercise
- Be able to interpret client feedback based on the nature of the questions and why they may affect program classification
- Be able to administer a Health Behavior Form and identify possible negative health behaviors

Activity 5.1 Heart Disease Risk Factors

Activity Description

Heart disease is the leading killer in the United States. It is well documented that a sedentary lifestyle, obesity, and poor nutritional habits accelerate the development of the disease. Personal trainers should be well-versed in the risk factors for heart disease and the behaviors linked to them. Exercise and routine physical activity along with healthy dietary habits and reduced stress exposure can help prevent the premature development of heart disease and thwart the cascade of events that may lead to a myocardial infarction or stroke.

Procedures

Connect the risk factors for heart disease with the resultant effect each has in the development of Coronary Artery Disease (CAD). There may be more than one negative effect for each risk factor. You may reference Chapter 12 for assistance if necessary.

Risk Factor for CAD	Negative Consequences
_____ High Blood Pressure	A. Increased LDL Cholesterol
_____ Low Grade Inflammation	B. Reduced HDL Cholesterol
_____ High Fat Diet	C. Reduced Adiponectin
_____ Saturated Fat	D. Increased Triglycerides
_____ Psychological Stress	E. Increased Platelet Adhesion
_____ Smoking	F. Endothelial Dysfunction/Damage
_____ Oxidative Stress (free radicals)	G. Endothelial Lesions
_____ Physical Inactivity	
_____ Visceral Fat	

Procedures

Order the cascade of events that leads to Coronary Artery Disease. Place a number next to the event in the order in which it occurs (1-15).

Cascade of CAD – Progression of Heart Disease

_____ LDL cholesterol deposits fat in the arterial wall

_____ Macrophages (immune cells) ingest fatty deposits

_____ Fibrotic cover develops between fat deposits and artery lining

_____ Blood clot formation

_____ Cellular ischemia – lack of oxygen

_____ Myocardial infarct – heart attack

_____ Inflammatory response

_____ Circulatory stress – turbulent blood flow

_____ Endothelial aneurysm

_____ Aneurysm rupture

_____ Endothelial lesion

_____ Circulatory material build-up in the vessel

_____ Occlusion/blockage

_____ Smooth muscle cell proliferation

_____ Development of collagen matrix – hardening of the vessel

Activity 5.2 Consent Form Administration

Activity Description

Prior to a person engaging in physical activity under the supervision of a personal trainer, there are several "clearance" procedures the trainer must initiate with the client in order to reduce the risk of liability in the event of a training accident or incident. Professional screening practices reduce trainer liability, foster communication with regard to the benefits and risks of physical activity, and ease client concern for exercise safety. The first of these procedures is the administration of an Informed Consent Form. The form serves several functions in the initial education of a client as to what to expect with exercise participation.

Exercise, as with all other forms of physical exertion, has some degree of risk. Although the risks for participation in an exercise program or testing protocol are relatively low, and whilst most health professionals believe that the benefits outweigh the risks, it is important for the personal trainer to ensure an optimal benefit-to-risk ratio. This requires that the risks are thoroughly explained to the client before engaging them in any mode of physical activity (including exercise testing).

From a legal standpoint, any participant involved in physical activity for which another party is responsible for the structure, prescription, organization, or assessment of the participant's actions must give informed consent for the exercise to be proper and lawful. Informed consent is intended to show that the participant entered into the activity or testing procedure with full knowledge of the procedures, relative risks, expected physiological occurrence, benefits, and alternatives, if applicable. To give valid consent, an individual must be of legal age and have all mental faculties. They must fully understand the importance and relevance of the material risks and provide a voluntary consent, preferably in writing, for increased legal protection. Written consent holds greater merit should questions to the procedure arise on a later occasion.

One of the fallacies regarding informed consent is that it relinquishes the person (trainer) from any and all responsibility in the event of an incident or training accident. This is not necessarily the case. Nothing will protect the trainer against liability stemming from trainer <u>negligence</u> (failing to explain and have the client sign a well written consent form is the first "negligent" thing a trainer can do). However, if the trainer has an informed consent document signed by the client which states the activities to be performed and the risks involved, the trainer can better protect themselves in the event of an incident. Additionally, the client accepts a level of accountability once they are made aware of the risks associated with the activities you wish to employ before they are undertaken. This allows them to make an educated and willful decision to participate.

Legal action arising from the informed consent procedure frequently occur when the injured party claims negligence based on the explanation or administration of the Informed Consent Form by the personal trainer. The result of the suit is often based on the informed consent process and the conduct by which the professional implemented the test or activity. This means that the informed consent must be as detailed as possible with regard to the exercises, assessments, and training procedures used, this includes modes, intensities, and possible health detriments (in some cases death). For example, if you will be utilizing free weights and other modes of resistance training, these should be listed in the consent form as well as the risks involved with their use.

From a communication standpoint, the trainer should explain the document and identify to the client that there are risks associated with the activity procedures and describe the measures to address specific concerns arising from the activity participation. This will create an open trainer/client relationship and assist in the education process for the client.

Procedures

The first formal step to getting a new client started in an exercise program is the administration of an Informed Consent Form. Using the steps highlighted below, administer the Informed Consent Form (provided) to a volunteer subject. After completing the administration of the document have a third party witness it to verify that the subject completely understands the information contained therein. Please keep this, as well as all volunteer subject information in a secure area. This is not only to maintain confidentiality, but the program requires you to have volunteer subjects perform physical activity under your supervision and it is wise to have this document signed and on file.

Step 1   *Purpose and explanation of the procedure.* Thoroughly explain all the activities the subject will be participating in, as well as the rationale behind the activity selection.

Step 2   *Explanation of risks.* Identify possible risks involved with basic exercise and the activities they will be participating in.

Step 3   *Explanation of benefits.* Explain the specific positive role the activity will play in developing their total fitness.

Step 4   *Procedures of the test or activity.* Provide clear instructions and timetables related to the activity so the subject knows exactly what to expect and has a good idea of what they will be doing.

Step 5   *Physiological expectations from the physical effort.* Identify the normal physical occurrences the subject may experience during the activity.

Step 6   *Explain confidentiality.* All information gathered during the test or activity is confidential.

Step 7   *Inquiries and freedom from consent.* Answer any questions the subject may have with regard to the activity and clearly state that they have the option to refuse participation.

Step 8   *Emergency contact information.* Although this is also provided on the Health Status Questionnaire (HSQ), it is beneficial to have this information in a readily accessible area.

INFORMED CONSENT

Purpose and Explanation of Service

I understand that the purpose of the exercise program is to develop and maintain healthy levels of cardiorespiratory fitness, body composition, flexibility, muscular strength and endurance. A specific exercise plan will be given to me, based on my needs and abilities. All exercise prescription components will comply with proper exercise program protocols. The programs include, but are not limited to, aerobic exercise, flexibility training, and strength training. All programs are designed to place a gradually increasing workload on the body in order to improve overall fitness.

Risks

I understand, and have been informed, that there exists the possibility of adverse changes when engaging in a physical activity program. I have been informed that these changes could include abnormal blood pressure, fainting, disorders of heart rhythm, stroke and very rare instances of heart attack or even death. I have been told that every effort will be made to minimize these occurrences by proper screening and by precautions and observations taken during the exercise session. I understand that there is a risk of injury, heart attack, or even death as a result of my participation in an exercise program, but knowing those risks, it is my desire to partake in the recommended activities.

Benefits

I understand that participation in an exercise program has many health related benefits. These may include improvements in body composition, range of motion, musculoskeletal strength and endurance, and cardiorespiratory efficiency. Furthermore, regular exercise can improve blood pressure and lipid profile, metabolic function, and decreases the risk of cardiovascular disease.

Physiological Experience

I have been informed that during my participation in the exercise program I will be asked to complete physical activities that may elicit physiological responses/symptoms that include, but are not limited to, the following: elevated heart rate, elevated blood pressure, sweating, fatigue, increased respiration, muscle soreness, cramping, and nausea.

Confidentiality and Use of Information

I have been informed that the information obtained in this exercise program will be treated as privileged and confidential and will not be released or revealed to any person without my express written consent. Any other information obtained, however, will be used only by the program staff to evaluate my exercise status as needed.

Inquiries and Freedom of Consent

I have been given an opportunity to ask questions about the exercise program. I further understand that there are also other remote health risks. Despite the fact that a complete accounting of all these remote risks has not been provided to me, I still desire to proceed with the exercise program. I acknowledge that I have read this document in its entirety or that it has been read to me if I have been unable to read same. I consent to the rendition of all services and procedures as explained herein by all program personnel.

_____

Date

_____

Participant Signature

_____

Witness Signature

_____

Trainer signature

Activity 5.3 Health Status Questionnaire

Activity Description
The second step in the screening process is to employ the use of a health appraisal tool prior to a participant engaging in physical activity. Administering a health appraisal to a new client prior to his or her participation in physical activity (exercise testing and any other form of physical activity) will: provide the personal trainer with information relevant to the safety of fitness testing before beginning exercise training; identify any known diseases and risk factors for coronary heart disease (CHD) and other potentially preventable chronic diseases; and identify additional factors that require special consideration in the development of an appropriate exercise prescription. This information allows the initiation of needed lifestyle interventions and exercise programming that will optimize adherence, minimize risks, and maximize benefits.

The Health Status Questionnaire (HSQ) is a widely used health appraisal tool for clearing participants into an exercise program. The HSQ is a four-part screening tool designed to provide the fitness professional with information about: any diagnosed medical problems, characteristics that increase the risk of health problems, signs or symptoms that increase the risk of health problems, and lifestyle behaviors related to positive or negative health. The HSQ is one of the first tools a personal trainer will employ prior to a client engaging in any form of physical activity under their supervision. The information provided on the HSQ can help to reduce trainer liability and is very beneficial in the creation of a comprehensive health profile of the prospective new client. The health profile is used to not only document and assess risk stratification, but also to help educate the client as to potential health problems stemming from lifestyle decisions, predisposed hereditary issues, and/or current medical conditions that can be positively affected by exercise.

The document is intended to be administered as an oral questionnaire. The rationale behind this method of implementation is to use the questions as probes for more information and greater detail about certain answers. Then, depending on the responses to the questions on the HSQ, the subject can be placed into one of three categories: medical referral, supervised program, or unrestricted activity. There are also specific action codes associated with many of the questions/responses to help the fitness professional choose a correct course of action when, and if, special procedures are necessary prior to beginning an exercise program. Knowing the correct course of action with regard to an individual's personal screening information is a vital aspect of the fitness professional's job description. Chapter 13 of your course textbook will provide you with further information pertaining to the specific criterion for classification.

Procedures
The following case study includes a completed HSQ document. Review the document and identify any responses related to the following: diagnosed medical problems, characteristics that increase the risk of health problems, signs or symptoms indicative of health problems, and lifestyle behaviors related to positive or negative health. You should also identify items that may positively or negatively affect the sample client's health and/or exercise program clearance.

Step 1   Review the HSQ document and identify significant and relevant findings.

Step 2   Stratify the risk by listing the findings in order of relevance and document the action codes for each.

Step 3   Analyze the findings and make a program participation decision for the sample subject.

Program participation recommendation _____

HEALTH STATUS QUESTIONNAIRE

SECTION ONE - GENERAL INFORMATION

1. Date: **7/6/2007**

2. Name: **John Delaney**

3. Mailing Address: **15 Elm St. Merribel, PA 18623**   Phone (H): **555-347-2830**

                                            Phone (W):

   Email: **JMoney@2times.com**

4. *EI* Personal Physician: **Dr. Vincent**   Phone:

   Physician Address: Fax:

5. *EI* Person to contact in case of emergency: **Mary Delaney**   Phone: **Same**

6. Gender (circle one): Female   **Male** *RF*

7. *RF* Date of birth: **06/23/65**

8. Height: **5'10"** Weight: **205**

9. Number of hours worked per week: Less than 20   20-40   **41-50**   over 50

10. *SLA* More than 25% of the time at your job is spent (circle all that apply):

     Sitting at desk   Lifting loads   Standing   Walking   Driving

SECTION TWO - CURRENT MEDICAL INFORMATION

11. Date of last medical physical exam: **06/14/2006**

12. Circle all medicine taken or prescribed within the last 6 months:

    Blood thinner *MC*   Epilepsy medication *SEP*   Nitroglycerin *MC*
    Diabetic *MC*   Heart rhythm medication *MC*   Other_____
    Digitalis *MC*   **High blood pressure medication** *MC*
    Diuretic *MC*   Insulin *MC*

13. Please list any orthopedic conditions. Include any injuries in the last six months.

        ACL tear in High School – Surgically repaired

14. Any of these health symptoms that occur frequently (two or more times/month) require medical attention. Please check any that apply.

a. ___ Cough up blood *MC*   g. ___ Swollen joints *MC*

b. ___ Abdominal pain *MC*   h. ___ Feel faint *MC*

c. ___ Low-back pain *MC*   i. ___ Dizziness *MC*

d. ___ Leg pain *MC*   j. ___ Breathlessness with slight exertion *MC*

e. ___ Arm or shoulder pain *MC*   k. ___ Palpitation or fast heart beat *MC*

f. ___ Chest pain *RF MC*   l. ___ Unusual fatigue with normal activity *MC*

Other_____

SECTION THREE - MEDICAL HISTORY

15. Please circle any of the following for which you have been diagnosed or treated by a physician or health professional:

Alcoholism *SEP*	Diabetes *SEP*	Kidney problem *MC*
Anemia, sickle cell *SEP*	Emphysema *SEP*	Mental illness *SEP*
Anemia, other *SEP*	Epilepsy *SEP*	Neck strain *SLA*
Asthma *SEP*	Eye problems *SLA*	Obesity *RF*
Back strain *SLA*	Gout *SLA*	Phlebitis *MC*
Bleeding trait *SEP*	Hearing loss *SLA*	Rheumatoid arthritis *SLA*
Bronchitis, chronic *SEP*	Heart problems *MC*	Stress *RF*
Stroke *MC*	Cancer *SEP*	**High blood pressure** *MC*
Thyroid problem *SEP*	Cirrhosis *MC*	HIV *SEP*
Ulcer *SEP*	Concussion *MC*	Hypoglycemia *SEP*
Congenital defect *SEP*	Hyperlipidemia *RF*	Other_____

16. Circle any operations that you have had:

Back *SLA*   Heart *MC*   Kidneys *SLA*   Eyes *SLA*   **Joints** *SLA*   Neck *SLA*

Ears *SLA*   Hernia *SLA*   Lungs *SLA*   Other_____

17. *RF* Circle any who died of heart attack before age 55:

Father   Brother   Son

18. *RF* Circle any who died of heart attack before age 65:

Mother   Sister   Daughter

SECTION FOUR - HEALTH-RELATED BEHAVIORS

19. Have you ever smoked?   Yes   **No**

20. *RF* Do you currently smoke? Yes   **No**

21. *RF* If you are a smoker, indicate the number smoked per day:

    Cigarettes: 40 or more   20-39   10-19   1-9

    Cigars or pipes only: 5 or more or any inhaled less than 5

22. *RF* Do you exercise regularly?   Yes   **No**

23. Last physical fitness test: **High School**

24. How many days a week do you accumulate 30 minutes of moderate activity?

                    0   1   2   3   4   5   6   7

25. How many days per week do you normally spend at least 20 minutes in vigorous exercise?

                    0   1   2   3   4   5   6   7

26. What activities do you engage in a least once per week?   **Golf**

27. Weight now: **205 lbs.**   One year ago: **200 lbs**.   Age 21:   **170 lbs.**

SECTION FIVE - HEALTH-RELATED ATTITUDES

28. These are traits that have been associated with coronary-prone behavior. Circle the number
    that corresponds to how you feel toward the following statement:

                I am an impatient, time-conscious, hard-driving individual.

                Circle the number that best describes how you feel:

        6= Strongly agree   3= Slightly disagree
        5= Moderately agree   2= Moderately disagree
        4= Slightly agree   1= Strongly disagree

29. How often do you experience "negative" stress from each of the following?

	Always	Usually	Frequently	Rarely	Never
Work:			X		
Home or family:				X	
Financial pressure:				X	
Social pressure:				X	
Personal health:				X	

30. List everything not included on this questionnaire that may cause you problems in a fitness test or fitness program.

_____

_____

_____

_____

Action Codes

EI = Emergency Information - must be readily available.

MC = Medical Clearance needed - do not allow exercise without physician's permission.

SEP = Special Emergency Procedures needed - do not let participant exercise alone; make sure the person's exercise partner knows what to do in case of an emergency.

RF = Risk Factor of CHD (educational materials and workshops needed).

SLA = Special or Limited Activities may be needed - you may need to include or exclude specific exercises.

Other (not marked) = Personal information that may be helpful for files or research.

Activity 5.4 Health Behavior Form

Activity Description

Identification of negative health behaviors and patterns is another important aspect of the personal trainer's role as a health provider. For optimal gains in health and fitness to take place, the client must not only engage in regular sustained physical activity, but also change detrimental dietary and behavioral habits. Although the Health Status Questionnaire provides the personal trainer with important health related information, it is still incomplete with regard to the development of a complete client health profile. Many health-related behaviors correlate with the findings on the HSQ. The Health Behavior Form can be utilized by the personal trainer to better identify problem areas and assist with client behavior modification.

Procedures

Review the following sample behavior form that coincides with the sample subject in the previous HSQ case study. Analyze the responses noting anything that may negatively affect his overall health status. After reviewing the behavior form, reference the HSQ noting any current conditions that may be affected by his or her behavior patterns.

Step 1   *Explain confidentiality.* Inform subject that all information given will be kept private and confidential.

Step 2   *Importance of accurate completion.* Explain the purpose of the Health Behavior Form and the importance of answering all questions as accurately as possible as they will affect program decisions.

Step 3   *Form administration.* Administer the Health Behavior Form to your subject by asking each question and recording the response.

Step 4   *Form review.* Review and evaluate the form to identify positive and negative behaviors that may affect current and future health status.

List positive and negative behaviors from the sample Behavior Questionnaire

Positive Behaviors   Negative Behaviors

_____   _____

_____   _____

_____   _____

Step 5   *Goal establishment.* Establish both short and long-term behavior modification goals.

Short-Term Goals

_____

_____

_____

Long-Term Goals

_____

_____

_____

Step 6   *Review and evaluate.* Analyze the Health Behavior Form and identify connecting factors between the behaviors and the documented health concerns found on the HSQ document.

Identify correlating factors from the HSQ and make recommendations.

Correlating Factor   Recommendations

1. _____   _____

                                              _____

2. _____   _____

                                              _____

3. _____   _____

                                              _____

BEHAVIOR QUESTIONNAIRE

1. How many servings of fruits and vegetables do you eat per day?
                              0   **1**   2   3+

2. How many caffeinated drinks (coffee, tea, cocoa, soft drinks) do you drink per day?
                              0   1-2   **3-4**   5+

3. How many glasses (8 ounces) of water do you drink per day?
                              0-3   **4-5**   6-7   8+

4. How many meals do you consume per day?
                              1-2   **3-4**   5-6   7+

5. I cook with and eat fats:
   ____   Nearly always cook/eat high fat foods (fried foods, shortening, butter, creams)
   ____   Cook/eat mostly high fat
   _X_   Cook/eat both high and low fat foods
   ____   Cook/eat mostly low fat
   ____   Cook/eat only low fat

6. My bread/grain eating habit is:
   ____   Nearly always eat refined (white bread, grains, rolls, crackers, cereal)
   ____   Eat mostly refined grain products
   _X_   Eat a mixture of refined and whole grain products
   ____   Eat primarily whole grain products
   ____   Eat only whole grain products

7. How often do you eat out:
         __X__   I eat out nearly every day
         _____   I eat out several times each week
         _____   I eat out a few times each month
         _____   I seldom or never eat out

8. My salty food habit is: (check all that apply)
         _____   I rarely eat salty foods (chips, pickles, soups, added salt)
         __X__   Occasionally I eat salty foods
         _____   I regularly eat salty food
         _____   I add salt to the foods I eat

9. During the past 30 days, did you diet to lose weight or to keep from gaining weight?

               Yes   **No**

      If Yes Explain:_____

10. My high fat snack eating habit is:
         _____   I eat high fat snack foods (potato chips) 3 or more times daily
         _____   I eat high fat snacks once or twice daily
         __X__   I eat high fat snacks a few times each week
         _____   I rarely or never eat high fat snacks

11. How often do you eat red meat?
         _____   I eat red meat nearly every day
         __X__   I eat red meat several times each week
         _____   I eat red meat a few times each month
         _____   I seldom or never eat red meat

12. How often do you eat cookies, cakes, sweets?
         _____   I eat cookies, cakes, sweets nearly every day
         _____   I eat cookies, cakes, sweets several times each week
         __X__   I eat cookies, cakes, sweets a few times each month
         _____   I seldom or never eat cookies, cakes, sweets

13. How many alcoholic beverages do you consume per week?
                          0-3   4-5   **6-7**   8+

14. On average, I sleep _____ hours a night.
                        3-4   **5-6**   7-8   8+

15. Outside of work, what physical and/or social activities do you engage in?

     Play golf, go boating and fishing.

Activity 5.5 Initial Needs Analysis

Activity Description

The Health Status Questionnaire (HSQ) and the Behavior Questionnaire provide much more information than simply that needed to make a program participation decision. Findings on the document can identify components of the exercise prescription based on the activities that meet the specific need of the risk factor or health problem. These findings can be further supported by a resting battery of tests to quantify the actual level of need. Diseases such as obesity, hypertension, and diabetes have defined protocols that best correct or manage the disease. When the HSQ identifies a problem, the protocols that provide the solution should be included in the exercise prescription.

Procedures

Using the following case study, identify the correct prescription components to meet the sample client's needs. Once the disease or health risk has been identified, complete the table by recommending a type of exercise or activity.

Step 1   Identify and list the disease or health risk associated with the measured score or value of the sample client.

Name: Steve Murphy

Sex: Male

Age: 57

Evaluation Criteria	Score	Disease or Health Risk
Body fat:	26%	_____
Waist circumference:	104 cm	_____
Fasting blood glucose:	121 mg/dl	_____
Systolic blood pressure:	158 mmHg	_____
Diastolic blood pressure:	112 mmHg	_____
Resting heart rate:	75 beats $\cdot$ min^{-1}	_____

Step 2   Using the list created from Step 1 identify the appropriate type of exercise (i.e. aerobic training) and the general intensity recommended for the selected activity category.

Disease or Health Risk	Type of Exercise	Recommended Intensity
Example: Hyperlipidemia	Aerobic training	70%-80% VO$_2$max or highest tolerable level
_____	_____	_____
_____	_____	_____
_____	_____	_____
_____	_____	_____
_____	_____	_____
_____	_____	_____

Lab Five Submission Form – Health Appraisal & Screening Protocols

1. List three risk factors related to heart disease and identify how they impact the cascade of events for disease development.

    1. _____

    2. _____

    3. _____

2. True or False. Having a signed Informed Consent Form releases a trainer from liability stemming from negligence.

3. List the components of the informed consent.

    1. _____

    2. _____

    3. _____

    4. _____

    5. _____

4. Attach a photocopy of the Informed Consent Form you administered to a sample subject during the performance of Activity 5.2.

5. Mr. Delaney asks what the relevance of question 10 on the HSQ is to his health status. What is the appropriate response?

    _____

    _____

6. What sort of training modifications should be made when working with a person diagnosed with high blood pressure and taking blood pressure medication?

    _____

    _____

Lab Five Submission Form – Health Appraisal & Screening Protocols

7. What is the relevance of question 28 on the HSQ?

_____

_____

8. Why would it be important to know if Mr. Delaney cooks with oil, butter, or sauces?

_____

_____

9. What aerobic training intensity level is most appropriate for a hypertensive client?

           Low   Moderate   High

10. What is the diagnostic criteria for metabolic disease risk for waist circumference in males?

        _____ cm

        _____ inches

Lab Six
Fitness Testing

Lab Six corresponds to the following textbook reading:

Assessment of Physical Fitness   Chapter 14

Lab Description

Fitness testing is an integral part of individualizing exercise prescription so that the personal trainer can address the most important health and fitness needs of a client. As with any endeavor directed at improvement, the first steps are identifying the weaknesses and formulating a plan to transform the current problem into an acceptable alternative. In fitness, this usually means identifying physiological limitations and applying actions that will improve the current conditions. Fitness testing can identify the current level or status of a measurable physical component and provide information for rationale decisions on how to bring it to an acceptable level.

To effectively utilize test information for programming, the tests must be accurate and reliable. The adage of "garbage in = garbage out" is very applicable when talking about fitness data. If a person's test scores are not accurate, then their exercise prescription will likely reflect the inaccuracies through lack of effectiveness. To ensure that the data is correct, personal trainers can take steps to increase the potential for testing values to be true measures of the assessment. Strictly following protocol, testing and calibrating the equipment, knowing the test environment and controlling conditions, preparing the test subject appropriately, organizing data, and paying close attention to detail are just a few of the steps to quality data collection.

Accurate testing data provides information for program decisions, establishes baselines or starting points, allows for goal-based objectives, guides exercise selection, and allows the client to be tracked to assess program effectiveness. The type of assessment employed will be client-specific, based on their capabilities and related factors. This lab reviews exercise tests for aerobic and anaerobic fitness. Chapter 14 covers additional testing protocols, several of which can be found in detail within this manual.

Explored Procedures
- Fitness Testing Preparation Checklist
- Forestry Step Test
- One Mile Walk Test
- 1.5 Mile Run Test
- YMCA Bike Test
- Multi-repetition Strength Test
- Push-up Test
- Abdominal Curl-up Test

Lab Objectives
- Identify the role of fitness testing in client evaluation and exercise prescription
- Be able to administer a fitness test preparation checklist
- Understand the components of cardiorespiratory fitness and the application of VO$_2$max for exercise prescription
- Successfully administer/perform select cardiorespiratory fitness tests
- Evaluate results and make recommendations based on the findings
- Properly implement multi-repetition strength assessments and calculate a predicted 1RM value
- Properly administer a push-up and curl-up assessment for the evaluation of muscular endurance
- Successfully utilize assessment results to develop an exercise prescription that addresses each of the fitness components of the muscular system

Activity 6.1 Fitness Testing Preparation Checklist

A key component to validity is subject pre-test preparation. Preparing the subject for the test requires specific directions on what to do or not to do prior to engaging in the test activity. This means providing a detailed list to improve compliance with all test preparation protocols. A Fitness Testing Preparation Checklist is valuable in successful preparation and aids in the validity of test results. The list attempts to identify factors that may change the results of the test from their true value. Personal trainers must be able to distinguish factors that have no effect on test scores from ones that may create false data.

Procedures

Complete the following Fitness Test Checklist using a volunteer subject. If any particular aspect of the checklist identifies a factor that may affect the lab outcome, document it and take the necessary steps to correct the situation prior to testing.

Fitness Testing Preparation Checklist

Subject Preparation
1. Subject has completed the informed consent. ____
2. Subject has been screened and cleared for participation. ____
3. Subject has read and understands the test procedures. ____
4. Subject understands the starting and stopping procedures. ____
5. Subject knows the stop test indicators. ____
6. Subject understands what is expected for each stage of the test. ____
7. Subject has complied with all pre-test instructions concerning:
   A. Rest. ____
   B. Food. ____
   C. Beverage and hydration status. ____
   D. Drugs – including prescription, stimulants, depressants, alcohol, and tobacco. ____
   E. Appropriate attire. ____
8. Subject does not have illness or injury. ____
9. Subject is not fatigued, stressed, or anxious. ____
10. Subject is not on any medication (prescription or non-prescription). ____
11. Subject has participated in the proper warm-up procedures. ____

Tester Preparation
1. Test to be administered has been determined. ____
2. The protocols for administration are understood. ____
3. Equipment has been tested, calibrated, and is in good working order. ____
4. All necessary equipment, supplies, and recording sheets are ready. ____
5. The test environment is within acceptable limits for:
   A. Cleanliness. ____
   B. Temperature. ____
   C. Humidity. ____
   D. Noise. ____
6. The timing and sequence of testing are set. ____
7. The starting and stopping instructions are clear. ____
8. The subject has been prepared appropriately and meets all guidelines for testing. ____
9. The test atmosphere and environment are controlled. ____
10. Post test activities and responsibilities are set. ____
11. Emergency procedures are determined and understood. ____

Cardiorespiratory Fitness Testing

Cardiorespiratory fitness (CRF) may be defined as how efficiently the body extracts oxygen from inhaled air, transports it to the working muscles, and then utilizes it within the active cells. Cardiorespiratory assessment involves measuring or predicting VO_2max to determine the relative efficiency of the body to consume and use oxygen. The VO_2max value represents how much oxygen, per kilogram of bodyweight, the body can use on a cellular level per unit of time. It most often is expressed scientifically as ($ml \cdot kg^{-1} \cdot min^{-1}$) and calculated by multiplying cardiac output by (a–v)O_2 difference, the measured difference between the oxygen content of the arteries and the veins. The more blood that can be expelled by the heart and the more oxygen that can be extracted from the blood during systemic circulation, the greater the cardiorespiratory efficiency of the body.

There are many assessment protocols available to measure the cardiorespiratory fitness level of an individual. The protocols can be classified into two main categories: maximal VO_2 testing and submaximal VO_2 testing. Assessment protocols that are classified as maximal require the user to perform the assessment activity at a predetermined resistance and speed, or maximal exertion, until the activity cannot be continued due to fatigue, or the test time or distance is completed.

In contrast to VO_2max testing, submax VO_2 tests are more commonly used in most non-clinical fitness environments. Submax VO_2 assessments are a prediction of maximal oxygen consumption. The physiological rationale for their use focuses on the positive relationship between oxygen consumption, heart rate, and exercise. Protocols are designed to measure specific populations and much like tests for other fitness components should be matched to the client. Improperly matching fitness tests and clients often invalidate the test scores. The following activities include several variations of cardiorespiratory fitness assessments which cover a variety of population segments.

Activity 6.2 Forestry Step Test

Activity Description

One of the more common types of cardiorespiratory fitness field tests is the step test. In most cases, the tests last between 2-5 minutes, employing varying step-pace protocols. The tests are applicable for most apparently healthy persons because they require limited movement economy and can be performed in almost any setting. The exercise intensity is generally low enough for most persons to complete the prescribed duration of 5 minutes and high enough to sufficiently raise the heart rates of physically fit persons to get an accurate assessment of their VO_2max. However, the test may be too intense for individuals with an extremely low fitness level, those that are obese, and for many individuals over the age of 60.

The physiological rationale for the prediction of maximal oxygen consumption is based upon the positive relationship between oxygen consumption and exercise. As with oxygen consumption, heart rate is linearly related to exercise. This means that heart rate and oxygen consumption are directly related. Although heart rates are not measured during the performance of the Forestry Step Test, there is enough evidence to support a high relationship between estimated exercise heart rates and the actual exercise heart rate.

The advantages of the Forestry Step Test over tests using shorter durations of two or three minutes is that steady-state heart rate is attained with adequate aerobic contribution and the test can be utilized for multiple populations to predict a subject's VO_2max. Shorter duration step tests provide a classification of cardiorespiratory fitness, but do not provide a predictive value of VO_2. Additionally, the recovery heart rate is much easier to manage than tests that require heart rate assessment during the exercise performance.

Activity Equipment

- Metronome that will keep a cadence of 90 beats per minute
- Stop watch
- 40 cm (15.75 in) box for men
- 33 cm (13.0 in) box for women
- Scale for subject's body weight (taken fully clothed)
- Heart rate monitor (optional)
- NCSF Course Text

Procedures

The following activity requires you to administer the Forestry Step Test to a volunteer subject. Be sure to read through the entire lab prior to implementing this assessment.

Step 1   *Preparation.* Ensure that the subject:
1. Has signed a consent form and has been cleared to participate in activity
2. Has been checked for fitness preparation (checklist – part 1)
3. Is wearing appropriate clothing for the activity
4. Has performed a general warm-up

Step 2   *Stop Test Indicators.* Read and explain the following Stop Test Indicators to the subject.

Indications to stop the test

- Subject no longer feels comfortable performing the test
- Subject's skin becomes pale
- Subject fails to keep cadence for 20 seconds or more
- Subject has an inability to focus attention
- Subject experiences faintness, dizziness, or light-headedness
- Subject experiences upset stomach or vomiting symptoms
- Subject experiences dysfunction in breathing
- Subject experiences chest pain
- Subject experiences side stitch, cramp, strain, or unusual fatigue

Step 3   *Practice Stepping.* Skill acquisition is an important aspect to ensuring test validity and reliability. The subject must be comfortable and proficient at performing the assessment criterion, otherwise the test should not be performed until the movement skill is mastered or another assessment protocol should be used in its place. The Forestry Step Test requires the use of a metronome set at 90 tones per minute. For every tone, the subject must either step up or step down.

Once the metronome is operating at the 90 tones per minute rate, have the subject face the appropriate sized step, (40 cm) for men and (33 cm) for women, and instruct him or her to practice stepping up and down on the box or step using the following four-count cadence.

"Up-one"	Foot #1 goes to the top of the step
"Up-two"	The other foot (#2) follows to the top of the step
"Down-one"	Foot #1 descends to the floor
"Down-two"	Foot #2 descends to the floor

After the subject is able to successfully step up and down on the box or step at the correct cadence (usually about 30 seconds), have them sit for 2-3 minutes. This will allow the elevation in heart rate from the skill acquisition period to return to resting state.

Step 4   *Begin Assessment.* Start the metronome at the correct 90 tone per minute cadence. Have the subject face the box and begin stepping whenever they feel comfortable. As soon as the subject takes the first step, the administrator should begin timing the assessment.

Clock time 0:00 - begin stepping

Step 5   *Test Performance.* Have subject continue stepping on and off the box, staying in exact accordance with the cadence for the full 5 minutes of the test. The test administrator should visually assess the client throughout the duration of the test for proper identification of any signs and symptoms that may require the test to be stopped (Step Test Indicators). The test administrator should also periodically ask the subject how they are feeling to assess the subject's relative rate of perceived exertion (RPE). The RPE for this type of submaximal assessment should not exceed 7 on a 1 to 10 scale or a 16 on a 1 to 20 scale.

Clock time 0:00 - 5:00 step test administration

Step 6   *Palpation Preparation.* When the stop watch reaches the five (5:00) minute mark have the subject stop stepping and sit down on the step. Be sure to keep the watch running as it will be used to assess the recovery heart rate of the subject. Locate the subject's radial pulse as the clock continues to run.

Clock time 5:00 - subject stops stepping and administrator palpates the radial pulse

Step 7   *Recovery Heart Rate Palpation.* Once the stopwatch reads 5:15 the test administrator should begin counting the subject's recovery heart rate through the palpation of the radial artery. Monitoring of the subject's heart rate should start at the 5:15 mark and end at the 5:30 mark. This will provide the number of times the subject's heart has cycled in 15 seconds.

Clock time 5:15 - 5:30 count pulse rate

Step 8   Record the 15 second recovery heart rate and have subject perform a cool down.

Pulse rate for 15 seconds =_____

Reasons for a Cool Down

It is important to perform a thorough cool down after exercise. Benefits of a cool down include acclimated restoration of the resting metabolism, the maintenance of cardiac output due to venous return, prevention of blood pooling, prevention of rapid drop of blood pressure, reduction in risk of delayed onset muscle soreness (DOMS), and a reduction in incidences of cramping. To avoid these symptoms it is best to walk around for about 3-5 minutes immediately following the test. After walking you should perform a comprehensive flexibility routine focusing on the muscle groups involved in the activity.

Procedures for Estimating VO$_2$Max

Step 1   *Calculate fitness level score.* Using the 15 second recovery heart rate recorded in Step 8, find the subject's non-age-adjusted fitness score using table A located on pages 272-273 of your course textbook. Table A is actually two tables and includes the values for men and women so it is important to refer to the correct gender table. Follow the left-hand column down until you find the number that represents the subject's 15 second recovery heart rate from Step 8. Follow the row over to the right until it intersects with the subject's weight found across the bottom of the chart. This number will provide you with the subject's non-age-adjusted fitness score.

Enter score here_____non-adjusted fitness score (**ml • kg^{-1} • min^{-1}**)

Step 2   *Calculate age-adjusted estimated VO$_2$max.* To find the age-adjusted fitness score you will need the value from Step 1. Identify the subject's fitness score on the top column of the table labeled Age-Adjusted Fitness Score (Table B) located on pages 273-274 of your course textbook. Match this score with the closest age value provided by the subject. This will provide the subject's age-adjusted fitness level or predicted VO$_2$max (ml • kg^{-1} • min^{-1}).

Enter score here_____age-adjusted fitness score (**ml • kg^{-1} • min^{-1}**)

Step 3   *Evaluating the Results.* To find out what fitness category the subject falls into refer to the table titled Aerobic Fitness Categories for Men and Women (Table C) located on page 274 of your course textbook. Match the subject's age in the left-hand column with the subject's age-adjusted fitness score from Step 2 (above).

Enter classification here_____

Activity 6.3 One Mile Walk Test

Activity Description

There is a variety of walking and running test protocols that a personal trainer can use to estimate the cardiorespiratory fitness of an individual. This manual explores field tests, as there are minimal equipment requirements necessary to perform the assessments. The tests can be performed in most environments and they accommodate individuals of varying ages and fitness levels.

Walking is a very basic human movement that the vast majority of the population can execute with relative ease. Running, on the other hand, is far more challenging for many adults. Run/walk field tests require the user to walk or run as fast as possible over a predetermined distance or for a predetermined period of time. They may be well suited for the apparently healthy client, but may not be appropriate for deconditioned individuals. Instead, subjects identified as extremely detrained should participate in a walking program for a few weeks prior to the performance of any assessment, as their cardiorespiratory fitness level is already (identifiably) too low.

Like other submax protocols, field tests for CRF rely on the correlation between submax workload and heart rates. The assessment capitalizes on the increased oxygen demand of the body to determine the fitness of an individual. The estimation of VO_2 relies on the average speed to complete the assessment and the heart rate response to the activity.

The One Mile Walk Test requires the subject to walk as fast as possible on a measured track or flat mile course. Heart rate is measured at the end of the test and this value is used to predict VO_2max (ml $\cdot$ kg^{-1} $\cdot$ min^{-1}). An additional benefit to this assessment is that it can be administered to a single subject or a group of subjects at the same time.

Procedures

The following activity involves administering the One Mile Walk Test on a volunteer subject. Be sure to read through the entire lab prior to implementing this assessment.

Step 1   *Preparation.* Ensure that the subject:
        1. Has signed a consent form and has been cleared to participate in activity
        2. Has been checked for fitness preparation (checklist – part 1)
        3. Is wearing appropriate clothes for activity
        4. Has performed a general warm-up

Step 2   *Stop Test Indicators.* Read and explain the following Stop Test Indicators to the subject.

Indications to stop the test:
- Subject no longer feels comfortable doing the test
- Subject's skin becomes pale
- Subject has an inability to focus attention
- Subject experiences faintness, dizziness, or light-headedness
- Subject experiences upset stomach or vomiting symptoms
- Subject experiences dysfunction in breathing
- Subject experiences chest pain
- Subject experiences side stitch, cramp, strain, or fatigue

Step 3   *Warm-Up*. Have subject warm-up by walking at a comfortable pace.

Step 4   *Stretch*. Have subject stretch thoroughly.

Step 5   *Review Procedures*. Explain the test protocol and answer any questions.

Step 6   *Test Start*. Have subject ready him or herself behind the beginning mark of the measured mile. Timer says "Ready, Go," and starts the watch as the subject begins walking, as fast as possible, the measured course. You may want to provide the time at each lap, as well as encouragement of effort to enhance test validity.

Step 7   *Test Finish*. At the end of the measured mile (4 laps on standard track) you call out the time to the subject as they cross the measured mile marker and record the number below.

One mile walk time_____

Step 8   *Palpate Heart Rate*. At the conclusion of the walk test immediately assess the subject's pulse for a **10 second** duration. A ten second heart rate is used to more accurately assess the actual heart rate during the activity, as the heart rate will decline as soon as the activity is stopped (end of test).

10 second heart rate_____ beats

Step 9   *Recording*. After recording the subject's 10 second heart rate, calculate the subject's 60 second heart rate by multiplying the 10 second value by 6.

10 second heart rate_____ x 6 = _____beats • min^{-1}

Step 10   *Cool down*. Have the subject perform a cool down (cool down procedures are outlined in the Forestry Step Test Lab).

Procedures for Estimating VO$_2$max

Step 1   *Organize Data*. To calculate the subject's fitness level (VO$_2$) you will need to have the subject or client's age, current body weight, and gender (this information should have already been gathered during the initial screening process). The information gathered from the performance of the test should be transferred to the following data-recording sheet.

Age	Weight	Gender	One Mile Walk Time	Calculated 60 sec. HR (Step 9)

Step 2   *Calculating Fitness Level*. The following formula is used to calculate VO$_2$max (ml • kg^{-1} • min^{-1}) for the One Mile Walk Test from the recorded information. Using the equation template that follows, calculate the estimated VO$_2$.

Calculating VO₂max

$$VO_2max \ (ml \cdot kg^{-1} \cdot min^{-1}) = 132.853 - 0.0769(weight) - 0.3877(age) + 6.315(gender) - 3.2649(time) - 0.1565(HR)$$

- Weight is in pounds
- Age is in years
- Gender = 0 for females and 1 for males
- Time is in minutes and hundredths of minutes (ex. 13.51 = 13 minutes and 31 seconds) *divide 31 seconds by 60 seconds*
- Heart rate is in beats per minute

0.0769 x _____ lbs = _____ Value #1

0.3877 x _____ years = _____ Value #2

6.3150 x _____ gender = _____ Value #3

3.2649 x _____ min. = _____ Value #4

0.1565 x _____ HR = _____ Value #5

132.853 – (Value #1) – (Value #2) + (Value #3) – (Value #4) – (Value #5) = _____ ml $\cdot$ kg^{-1} $\cdot$ min^{-1}

In the space provided, calculate the subject's estimated VO₂max (ml $\cdot$ kg^{-1} $\cdot$ min^{-1}) from the One Mile Walk Test results.

132.853 – (_____ #1) – (_____ #2) + (_____ #3) – (_____ #4) – (_____ #5) = _____ ml $\cdot$ kg^{-1} $\cdot$ min^{-1}

Predicted VO₂max _____ ml $\cdot$ kg^{-1} $\cdot$ min^{-1}

Activity 6.4 1.5 Mile Run Test Assessment

Activity Description

Similar to the One Mile Walk Test, the administration protocols for the 1.5 Mile Run Test requires the subject to travel a timed distance to predict VO₂max . This assessment calls for the subject to jog/run 1.5 miles as fast as possible on a measured track. The total time used to complete the distance is converted into an estimated VO₂max using calculations. Like the walk test, this assessment can be administered to a single subject or a group of subjects at the same time. A major difference between walking and running tests is the role effort plays in the test outcome. Individuals that do not put forth a maximal effort will receive a score that under predicts their actual oxygen efficiency. Additionally, running tests are used for healthy individuals with previous running experience. New exercisers should avoid maximal run tests as their risk for a negative outcome is elevated and the data will likely skew due to poor economy and pacing.

Procedures

The following activity requires the administration of the 1.5 Mile Run Test to a test subject. Be sure to read through the entire lab prior to implementing this assessment.

Step 1   *Preparation.* Ensure that the subject:

                1. Has signed a consent form and has been cleared to participate in activity

                2. Has been checked for fitness preparation (checklist – part 1)

                3. Is wearing appropriate clothes for activity

                4. Has performed a general warm-up

Step 2   *Stop Test Indicators.* Read and explain the following Stop Test Indicators to the subject.

Indications to stop the test:

- Subject no longer feels comfortable doing the test
- Subject's skin becomes pale
- Subject has an inability to focus attention
- Subject experiences faintness, dizziness, or light-headedness
- Subject experiences upset stomach or vomiting symptoms
- Subject experiences dysfunction in breathing
- Subject experiences chest pain
- Subject experiences side stitch, cramp, strain, or fatigue

Step 3   *Warm-Up.* Have subject warm-up with some slow jogging.

Step 4   *Stretch.* Have subject stretch thoroughly.

Step 5   *Review Procedures.* Explain the purpose of the test to the test subject and answer any questions they may have regarding the procedure. Clearly inform the test subject that they are to run/jog 6 laps (1.5 miles standard track) or the full distance of the course as fast as possible.

Step 6   *Test Prep.* Have the test subject stand behind the starting line of the measured distance.

Step 7   *Test Start.* Timer says "Ready, Go" and starts the stop watch as the test subject begins running the 1.5 mile distance (6 laps on standard track).

Step 8   *Monitor.* When the test subject passes the start/stop line, inform him or her of the lap number they are on and the time. Look for signs of physical distress throughout the duration of the test.

Step 9   *Test Finish.* At the completion of lap 6, or 1.5 miles, the timer calls out the participant's time and records it.

Record 1.5 mile run time here_____

Procedures for Estimating VO₂max

Step 1   *Review of Formula.* Calculating the fitness level (estimated VO_2max) from the subject's 1.5 mile run time involves the use of the following formula:

$$VO_2 = \text{horizontal velocity } m \cdot min^{-1} \times \frac{0.2\ ml \cdot kg^{-1} \cdot min^{-1}}{m \cdot min^{-1}} + 3.5\ ml \cdot kg^{-1} \cdot min^{-1}$$

Step 2   *Finding horizontal run speed in (m · min⁻¹).* The formula is not as complicated as it appears. The first thing that must be determined is the average horizontal running velocity of the subject in meters per minute. To do this you must convert the distance completed into meters and divide it by the number of minutes it took to complete the full distance.

Example Meter Conversion
1.5 miles = 2,413.8 meters
2,413.8 must then be divided by the time it took to complete the run in minutes (use whole numbers)

Example (m • min^{-1}) conversion

12:00 minutes to complete the run

2,413.8 m / 12 min. = 201.15 m $\cdot$ min^{-1} (horizontal velocity)

If it took 12:13 to complete the run, the divisor would be 12.21 (12 +13/60))

Perform your conversion below:

2,413.8 meters ÷ _____ minutes = _____ m $\cdot$ min^{-1} (horizontal velocity)

Step 3   *VO_2max Conversion.* Calculate the subject's estimated VO_2max. Consider the above example:

Example VO_2max conversion

$$VO_2 = \text{horizontal velocity m} \cdot \text{min}^{-1} \times \frac{0.2 \text{ ml} \cdot \text{kg}^{-1} \cdot \text{min}^{-1}}{\text{m} \cdot \text{min}^{-1}} + 3.5 \text{ ml} \cdot \text{kg}^{-1} \cdot \text{min}^{-1}$$

$$VO_2 = 201 \text{ m} \cdot \text{min}^{-1} \times \frac{0.2 \text{ ml} \cdot \text{kg}^{-1} \cdot \text{min}^{-1}}{\text{m} \cdot \text{min}^{-1}} + 3.5 \text{ ml} \cdot \text{kg}^{-1} \cdot \text{min}^{-1}$$

$$VO_2 = 43.7 \text{ ml} \cdot \text{kg}^{-1} \cdot \text{min}^{-1}$$

Perform your conversion below:

$$VO_2 = \underline{\hspace{2cm}} \text{ horizontal velocity m} \cdot \text{min}^{-1} \times \frac{0.2 \text{ ml} \cdot \text{kg}^{-1} \cdot \text{min}^{-1}}{\text{m} \cdot \text{min}^{-1}} + 3.5 \text{ ml} \cdot \text{kg}^{-1} \cdot \text{min}^{-1}$$

$$VO_2 = \underline{\hspace{2cm}} \text{ ml} \cdot \text{kg}^{-1} \cdot \text{min}^{-1}$$

The following chart can also be used as a quick reference

1.5 Mile Time	VO_2max ml $\cdot$ kg^{-1} $\cdot$ min^{-1}	1.5 Mile Time	VO_2 max ml $\cdot$ kg^{-1} $\cdot$ min^{-1}
<7:31	75	12:31 – 13:00	39
7:31 – 8:00	72	13:01 – 13:30	37
8:01 – 8:30	67	13:31 – 14:00	36
8:31 – 9:00	62	14:01 – 14:30	34
9:01 – 9:30	58	14:31 – 15:00	33
9:31 – 10:00	55	15:01 – 15:30	31
10:01 – 10:30	52	15:31 – 16:00	30
10:31 – 11:00	49	16:01 – 16:30	28
11:01 – 11:30	46	16:31 – 17:00	27
11:31 – 12:00	44	17:01 – 17:30	26
12:01 – 12:30	41	17:31 – 18:00	25

Adapted from Adams

Activity 6.5 YMCA Bike Test

Activity Description

Cycle ergometry is a very popular fitness assessment tool for several obvious reasons: 1) It offers relatively easy implementation in most environments due to the portable, moderate cost instrumentation, 2) The movement performance is easily learned in a short period of time with limited loss to economy, reducing the skill acquisition period, 3) The standardized revolutions make it easy to control effort and the fact that the exercise is non-weight bearing gives it merit with populations where orthopedic limitations are a concern. Some concern does arise with regards to leg muscle fatigue. This is of particular interest when making decisions for aerobic testing in different population segments. If the test becomes invalid due to leg fatigue, an alternative test should be selected in its place.

The YMCA Bike Test is a multi-stage assessment requiring the user to pedal at a predetermined rate. The resistance is then increased (power output) according to the heart rate response at the given workload. Each stage of the test lasts approximately 3 minutes unless the subject has not reached a steady-state heart rate during the stage. Remember that steady-state heart rate is defined as a change (+ or -) of no greater the 5 beats $\cdot$ min^{-1}. If an individual reaches the end of the three minutes without reaching steady-state heart rate, the stage is extended another minute. During the entire test the pedal rate is maintained at 50 revolutions per minute (50 rev $\cdot$ min^{-1}). This is necessary to maintain a constant variable for workload calculation. Using a Monarch Cycle Ergometer, a .5 kp increase in resistance is equal to 150 kgm $\cdot$ min^{-1} when revolutions are maintained at the designated constant. Seat height is adjusted so that the maximum knee extension on the downward stroke is 5 degrees (slightly bent). Heart rate is measured and recorded during the latter half of the second and third minutes of each stage.

There are several factors to take into consideration when using cycle ergometer tests to estimate VO$_2$max. The most important of which is the initial work rate and the rate of progression through the stages. Body weight, sex, age, and current fitness level all may influence the initial work rate and progression of the test. In general, absolute VO$_2$max (L $\cdot$ min^{-1}) is lower in smaller people, women have lower absolute VO$_2$max values than men, VO$_2$max decreases with age, and inactivity is associated with a low VO$_2$max. The YMCA test addresses these issues by starting all subjects at a workload of 150 kgm $\cdot$ min^{-1} and using the heart rate response of each stage to set the subsequent workload.

Activity Equipment

- Cycle ergometer (Monark 818E)
- Stop watch
- Metronome if bike is not equipped with a RPM indicator
- Blood pressure monitoring device
- Heart rate monitor (recommended)

Procedures

The following activity requires the administration of the YMCA Bike Test to a test subject. Be sure to read through the entire lab prior to implementing this assessment.

Test Preparation

- Review the previously outlined Stop Test Indicators
- Explain the procedures of the YMCA test to the subject
- Have the subject sign an Informed Consent Form
- Evaluate subject using the Fitness Preparation Checklist

Calculate subjects predicted heart rate max (220 - age)   _____ beats $\cdot$ min^{-1}

Calculate 85% of heart rate max   _____ beats $\cdot$ min^{-1}

Set the seat height and record for retesting   _____

- If an RPM indicator is not available, start the metronome (set at 100 beats $\cdot$ min^{-1}) so that one foot is at the bottom of the pedaling stroke on each beat. This will result in the required 50 rev $\cdot$ min^{-1} for the entire test.

- Have the subject pedal for 30 seconds. This will allow for practice at maintaining proper intensity and allow the tester to set the cycle ergometer to the required resistance of 150 kgm $\cdot$ min^{-1} or .5 kp.

- Have the subject rest for 3 minutes following skill attainment and ensure the ergometer is set to the required resistance.

- Use the provided data recording sheet to assist you in tracking the results of each stage.

Step 1 (0:00 – 1:30)   *Test Start.* With the metronome running at the 100 beats $\cdot$ min^{-1} cadence, start the timer as soon as the subject begins pedaling at the required 50 rev $\cdot$ min^{-1} using first stage work rate of 150 kgm $\cdot$ min^{-1} (.5 kp).

Step 2 (1:30)   *Monitor Blood Pressure.* Take and record subject's blood pressure (see recording sheet).

Step 3 (2:00)   *Monitor Heart Rate.* Take and record subject's heart rate (see recording sheet).

Step 4 (2:50)   *Assess RPE.* Ask participant how they are feeling and record subject's RPE (see recording sheet).

Step 5 (3:00)   *Monitor Heart Rate Response to Determine Subsequent Workload.* Take and record the subject's heart rate. If subject's heart rate is less than the 85% of max, blood pressure is responding normally, and the participant is performing to protocol satisfaction, increase the resistance to the next stage. Refer to the table below to find out the correct workload for the next stage setting. The subsequent workloads are based on the heart rate responses at the end of each stage.

Step 6   Repeat steps 1-5 increasing workload by the correct increments until a steady-state heart rate of over 110 beats $\cdot$ min^{-1} is attained. The subject should then continue one more stage after a heart rate of 110 beats $\cdot$ min^{-1} is reached. For example, if during stage 2 the subject's 2nd minute heart rate is 113 beats $\cdot$ min^{-1} and 3rd minute heart rate is 115 beats $\cdot$ min^{-1} then they have reached steady-state and also have reached the desired 110 beats $\cdot$ min^{-1} for the test. The instructor should then have the subject proceed with one more stage following the outlined workload protocols below and record all designated physiological values on the provided chart.

Step 7   Plot results from each stage on the graph on the following page.

**Be sure to extend any stage by one minute if a steady state heart rate is not reached by the end of the third minute within the respective stage.

Time	Stagee	Heart Rate Response and Corresponding Workload			
0:00-3:00	1st	150 kgm $\cdot$ min^{-1}			
3:00-6:00	2nd	HR <80 750 kgm	HR 80-89 600 kgm	HR 90-100 450 kgm	HR >100 300 kgm
6:00-9:00	3rd	HR <80 900 kgm	HR 80-89 750 kgm	HR 90-100 600 kgm	HR >100 450 kgm
9:00-12:00	4th	HR <80 1050 kgm	HR 80-89 900 kgm	HR 90-100 750 kgm	HR >100 600 kgm

YMCA Data Recording Sheet

Name:		Sex:	Age:	Weight:	Max HR:	85% HR:
Stage 1	150 kgm · min⁻¹	150 kgm · min⁻¹	150 kgm · min⁻¹	150 kgm · min⁻¹	150 kgm · min⁻¹
0:00-3:00	2nd min HR	3rd min HR	Steady state	1:30 BP mmHg	RPE:1-10
			Y or N		
Stage 2	_____ kgm · min⁻¹	_____ kgm · min⁻¹	_____ kgm · min⁻¹	_____ kgm · min⁻¹	_____ kgm · min⁻¹
3:00-6:00	2nd min HR	3rd min HR	Steady state	1:30 BP mmHg	RPE:1-10
			Y or N		
Stage 3	_____ kgm · min⁻¹	_____ kgm · min⁻¹	_____ kgm · min⁻¹	_____ kgm · min⁻¹	_____ kgm · min⁻¹
6:00-9:00	2nd min HR	3rd min HR	Steady state	1:30 BP mmHg	RPE:1-10
			Y or N		
Stage 4	_____ kgm · min⁻¹	_____ kgm · min⁻¹	_____ kgm · min⁻¹	_____ kgm · min⁻¹	_____ kgm · min⁻¹
9:00-12:00	2nd min HR	3rd min HR	Steady state	1:30 BP mmHg	RPE:1-10
			Y or N		

Plot subject's 3rd minute Heart Rate response at each of the given workloads

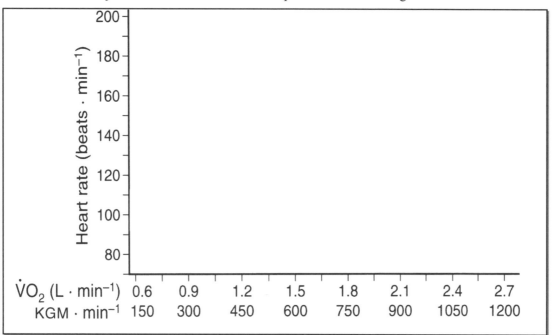

Step 8   After plotting the heart rate values at the completion of the 2nd or 3rd workloads, extrapolate the line outward to the subject's age-predicted maximum heart rate. Then draw a line downward toward the x-axis. Where the line bisects the x-axis is the subject's predicted VO_2 max.

Step 9   Record the predicted VO_2 max value _____ $L \cdot min^{-1}$

Step 10   Convert to relative VO_2 max _____ $ml \cdot kg^{-1} \cdot min^{-1}$

Sample Subject
40 year-old male, previously sedentary, no contraindications to exercise

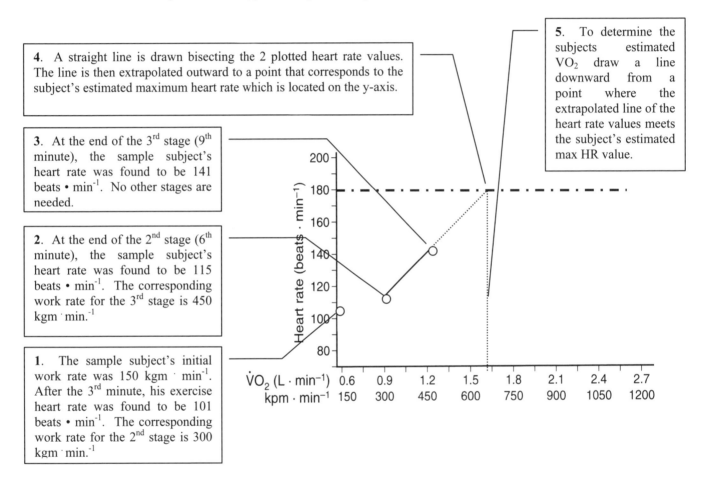

4. A straight line is drawn bisecting the 2 plotted heart rate values. The line is then extrapolated outward to a point that corresponds to the subject's estimated maximum heart rate which is located on the y-axis.

5. To determine the subjects estimated VO_2 draw a line downward from a point where the extrapolated line of the heart rate values meets the subject's estimated max HR value.

3. At the end of the 3rd stage (9th minute), the sample subject's heart rate was found to be 141 beats • min^{-1}. No other stages are needed.

2. At the end of the 2nd stage (6th minute), the sample subject's heart rate was found to be 115 beats • min^{-1}. The corresponding work rate for the 3rd stage is 450 kgm • $min.^{-1}$

1. The sample subject's initial work rate was 150 kgm • min^{-1}. After the 3rd minute, his exercise heart rate was found to be 101 beats • min^{-1}. The corresponding work rate for the 2nd stage is 300 kgm • $min.^{-1}$

Anaerobic (Muscular) Strength Assessments

Muscular strength and endurance are two of the five health-related components of fitness. The body requires adequate levels of both muscular strength and endurance in order to maintain proper locomotive function and joint health. Unfortunately, due to increasingly sedentary lifestyles, many people are not maintaining adequate physical activity levels, and therefore are not maintaining adequate levels of anaerobic strength and endurance over their lifespan. Many injuries and ailments that affect human performance and function can be attributed to poor muscular strength and endurance including postural and peripheral stabilization. Additionally, strength imbalances can affect proper joint function as stress is produced from uneven force couples. One of the responsibilities of a personal trainer is to assess, condition, and monitor client muscular strength and endurance and make proper program determinations/modifications based on findings, performance results, goals, and client feedback.

Muscle strength can be defined as the force that a muscle or muscle group can voluntarily exert against a resistance in one maximal effort. There is no formula for strength as the force produced by the body can occur without a velocity or speed component or require any joint movement as seen in isometric contractions. Lack of consistent muscular activity is the main reason strength declines. As muscles atrophy, strength decreases to a point that may compromise the ability to perform normal tasks. Loss of strength and power are associated with loss of function and independence.

Assessing muscular strength is a fundamental aspect to proper program prescription and modification. Initial training load and subsequent training prescription details should reflect the results of muscular strength assessments. Although muscular strength is defined as the force that a muscle or muscle group can voluntarily exert against a resistance in one maximal effort, it is often neither safe nor practical to have a client perform a one repetition maximum (1RM) assessment. Instead, a 1RM can be estimated through a formula based upon the successful number of completed repetitions using a submaximal load. Strength assessment using multiple repetition tests are commonly performed on cross joint movements such as the squat, deadlift, leg press, row, and press. The cross joint assessment increases the use of stabilization from contributing musculature which often is the determining factor in maximal force output when performing free or non-machine movements.

Activity 6.6 Multi-Repetition Bench Press

Activity Description
Repetition testing can be a safe and effective way to evaluate and monitor strength gains. Although it does not require a person to perform a 1RM, there is a close relationship between the amount of weight a person can lift one time and the amount of weight that they can lift a few times. To maintain a high correlation between 1RM and multi-repetition predictions the strength tests should be limited to no more than 10 repetitions and no fewer than 3 repetitions. Staying within this range will help ensure safety and test validity.

The following activity will have you perform a repetition test using the free weight bench press to determine a 1RM for a test subject. The assessment protocols can be applied to any number of free weight or machine resistance movements and are valuable to predict training intensities as well as track and monitor program effectiveness. The bench press is chosen for this activity because it is a good indicator of overall upper body strength as it involves the synergistic actions of shoulder horizontal adduction and arm extension. Additionally, because it is a free weight movement, it calls upon the stabilizing properties of the associated musculature.

The accuracy of strength testing is subject to several factors. The primary factor is the role of the nervous system. Since the performance of maximal muscle contractions is nervous system dependent, it is important to consider emotional and mental factors before performing tests to assess muscular strength. Other factors which may be considered include daily fatigue, energy system capacity, and hydration status. In tests requiring short duration and maximal contractions, blood supply is not a limiting factor because the role of oxygen is de-emphasized during energy metabolism for short burst activities.

It is important to note that if a person is new to exercise, strength testing, albeit free weight or machine, may be unwarranted until a baseline of strength, stability, and movement proficiency is developed. This can take a few sessions to acquire. You may also want to avoid exposing a person to such high physical demands if they have never performed resistance training before. This may have a deterrent effect for future resistance training participation if they experience a high degree of soreness from the assessment.

Activity Equipment

- Free weight bench press
- 45 lb. Olympic bar – if an individual cannot lift 45 lbs. lighter bars can be substituted
- Adequate free weight
- Safety clips

Procedures

Strength is measured using units of force or torque. These units may be expressed as pounds (lbs.), kilograms (kg), or newtons (N). For this lab we will be using pounds as the unit of force.

Prior to testing, determine a weight that can be lifted for approximately five repetitions. If an individual cannot perform at least 15 modified push-ups (female) or 20 conventional push-ups (male), they should not use this test. In addition, the test should not be used if it is the first time the subject has performed the bench press technique.

Step 1	*Warm-up.* Make sure that the subject has performed an adequate warm-up and is prepared for the test, using the test preparation checklist. The technician should always inspect the equipment prior to each test to be sure it is in proper working condition.
Step 2	*Protocol Review.* (Review Steps #3 – #6) Have the test subject perform two or three low intensity trials to make sure his or her form is perfect and that the subject is comfortable with the equipment. This will also act as a specific warm-up, increasing neural preparation and movement efficiency.
Step 3	*Ready Position.* Have the individual lie in the supine position on a flat bench with feet flat on the floor. Be sure the body lines up appropriately with the bench. The subject should not be too far forward or too far back on the bench (normal alignment is eyes under the bar). The technician should be directly behind the bar, attentive, and in a position to manage the bar movement.
Step 4	*Lift Off.* Instruct the subject to signal you when he or she is ready to lift the bar. Have them lift the bar off the rack while you assist. Their arms should be fully extended with the bar positioned over the chest. Instruct the subject to maintain the starting position as you release support on the bar.
Step 5	*Downward Movement Phase.* In the eccentric movement phase, the subject lowers the bar to his or her chest in a controlled manner. Instruct the subject to maintain strict body position and to keep the wrists straight. Once the bar makes contact with the chest, or the terminal ROM is reached, the subject's wrists should be directly over their elbows.
Step 6	*Upward Movement Phase.* In the concentric phase movement, the subject pushes the bar upward to full elbow extension. Instruct them to maintain body position without arching the back or lifting the glutes off the bench. Be sure the subject pushes the bar up evenly.
Step 7	*Movement Repetition.* Repeat steps 5 and 6 (downward and upward movement phases) until muscular failure is reached and the subject cannot complete another repetition. Safely re-rack the bar and then record results on the Data Recording Sheet.

*** Danger ***

It is important to closely monitor each repetition for volitional fatigue or poor body mechanics. If the individual shows signs of stability fatigue or an inability to maintain posture – stop the test. Also, be sure the subject is breathing correctly during each repetition, inhaling during the eccentric and exhaling during the concentric movement.

Step 8   *Calculate 1RM from Results.* Using the formula below, calculate the estimated 1RM using the weight lifted and the number of repetitions completed. Record results on data recording form.

Example

A male performs 5 repetitions to failure using 150 lbs.

3% Formula

[(0.03 x repetitions attained) + 1.0] x weight used

Estimated 1RM = [(0.03 x 5 repetitions) + 1.0] x 150 lbs.

Estimated 1RM = 1.15 x 150 = 172.5 lb

Multi-Repetition Strength Data Recording Form

Name: _____   Date: _____

Gender: _____   Age: _____   Body Weight: _____ lb. _____ kg

Exercise/Movement Assessed: _____

Resistance used: _____ lb.   Repetitions: _____

Multi-Repetition Formula

[(0.03 x repetitions performed _____) + 1.0] x weight used _____ lb.

[_____ + 1.0] x _____ lb.

Bench Press Score = _____ lb.

Step 9   *Interpret Results.* The table that follows illustrates Relative Bench Press Strength Norms based on body weight in both males and females. To find your subject's strength classification divide the subject's calculated 1RM by his or her current body weight.

Weight lifted ÷ body weight = upper body strength rating

_____ weight lifted ÷ _____ body weight = _____ upper body strength rating

Upper Body Strength Rating _____

Relative Bench Press Strength Norms

Classification	20-29 Y		30-39 Y		40-49 Y		50-59 Y		60 + Y	
	M	F	M	F	M	F	M	F	M	F
Above Average	>1.17	>.72	>1.01	>.62	>.91	>.57	>.81	>.51	>.74	>.51
Average	.97-1.16	.59-.71	.86-1.00	.53-.61	.78-.90	.48-.56	.70-.80	.43-.50	.63-.73	.41-.50
Below Average	<.96	<.58	<.85	<.52	<.77	<.47	<.69	<.42	<.62	<.40

Anaerobic (Muscular) Endurance Assessments

Muscular strength and endurance are interrelated, but differ in the amount of force produced to accomplish a task. Muscular endurance is defined as the ability of the muscle to contract repeatedly while resisting fatigue over a prolonged period of time. Often referred to as localized muscular endurance, the ability of a muscle to continue to produce force to maintain an activity is dependent upon the strength of the muscle itself, as well as the stabilizers that support the movement. Muscles that are weak do not maintain the ability to perform repetitive contractions when the force demands increase. This limits the ability of the body to perform beneficial activities and may become an obstacle to improving physical fitness.

Anaerobic muscle endurance is typically determined by a measured number of repetitions or by the ability to perform an activity at a set intensity for a predetermined period of time. It differs from aerobic endurance in the fact that 1) it emphasizes the anaerobic energy system 2) a person may have adequate cardiovascular conditioning, but may not be able to sustain localized muscular contractions due to rapid fatigue in the active musculature. It is also important to understand that both muscle strength and endurance are highly specific to the musculature being tested or trained. A high level of strength and/or endurance in a particular muscle, or group of muscles, does not translate to high levels of total muscular system endurance. Muscle endurance is muscle group specific in the same way flexibility is joint specific.

Several assessment protocols have been developed and are widely utilized in the fitness setting to assess anaerobic muscular endurance. Common examples include the push-up test, modified push-up test, and the abdominal curl-up test. These assessments are designed to address the unique characteristics of anaerobic muscular endurance in a specific region. They are often better tolerated by new exercisers due to the ease of execution and lower force production requirements to perform the movement.

Activity 6.7 Push-up Test / Modified Push-up Test

Activity Description

A very popular method to assess upper body endurance is the push-up test. It has classically been one of the primary field tests used to measure upper body endurance in individuals and groups. The test provides an accurate assessment of endurance if performed correctly. Therefore, it is extremely important for the test subject to adhere to proper movement technique, as the accuracy of testing and validity is negatively affected if correct form is not maintained. Many individuals do not possess the trunk strength to maintain the proper posture while performing the pressing movement from the ground. For this reason, the push-up test is often subject to tester discretion which can cause test validity to be skewed. To accurately assess anaerobic endurance capacity, each repetition must be performed with exacting technique throughout the duration of the test. The following procedures describe the test in detail.

Note: Although the push-up test is designed as an anaerobic endurance assessment, it can become a measure of anaerobic muscular strength when people do not possess the ability to perform multiple repetitions with proper form. When the test subject's muscles are only able to generate enough force to complete a few repetitions the test is actually identifying anaerobic strength rather than anaerobic endurance.

Procedures

The push-up test requires a subject to perform a maximal number of repetitions in the allotted time period. For this test, 60 seconds will be used. The subject may reach failure early in the test. If this occurs, they may rest in the starting position until they are able to perform additional repetitions. If an individual fails to perform the repetitions with the appropriate form, the test should be stopped. Other reasons for disqualification include failure to maintain body position or an inability to move the entire body through the required range of motion. Incorrect movements should not be scored. If the subject fails to perform the movement correctly for more than three repetitions, they should be asked to stop the test.

Prior to testing, the test subject should be instructed on proper movement technique. As in any exercise test, they should meet the pre-test requirements of the test checklist. Following an adequate warm-up, the subject should perform the technique for a minimum of 3-4 repetitions to insure that their ability and technique allow for safe testing procedures. If they cannot perform or are unable to follow the instructions listed below, they should not be tested using the assessment protocol.

The execution technique varies slightly for males and female. Be sure to read through each description and implement the proper gender specific assessment protocols.

Push-up (Males)

Step 1   *Test Setup.* Select an area with a solid, flat surface. Make sure that the area selected is in an environment that is safe and free of hazards. You may want to place a gym mat on the ground in an area that offers sufficient space for the assessment to be performed safely.

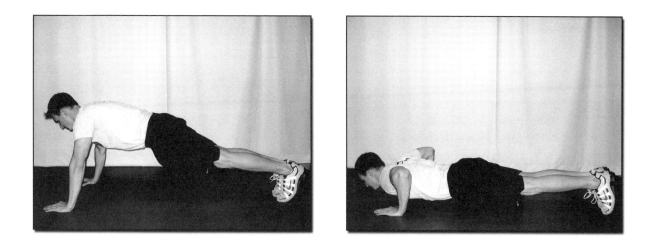

Step 2   *Starting Position.* Have the subject lie prone on the floor with his body extended. Place the hands approximately shoulders-width apart with thumbs located directly under the shoulders. The feet should be no more than 6" apart. Have the subject lift the body to a point where the arms are completely extended and the body is in proper alignment (do not allow the subject to perform hip extension or hip flexion during any phase of the movement).

Step 3   *Begin Assessment.* Once the subject is in position, the technician should give the "go" command and begin timing. The subject should lower themselves in a rigid straight position down to a point at which their elbows are at approximately 90° of flexion.

Step 4   *Movement Repetition.* The subject returns to the extended arm position by pushing upward until the elbows are fully extended. This movement should be performed until volitional failure, technique breakdown occurs, or the full 60 second duration of the test is completed. Count out loud each repetition the subject completes correctly.

Note: During the execution of the test be sure that the subject performs the movement through full ROM. It is common for a test subject to limit ROM during arm flexion and extension to try and achieve a higher score. It is also important that the subject maintains rigid body position. At no time should the spine/torso be placed in a flexed or hyperextended position.

Common mechanical performance errors to look for include:

- Excessive scapular protraction and retraction without adequate elbow flexion
- Scapular elevation
- Excessive humeral abduction
- Hip flexion or hip and back extension from lack of core strength
- Incorrect wrist to elbow relationship
- Incorrect hand placement including inward rotation

Step 5   *Data Collection/Recording.* Record the number of repetitions successfully performed in one minute on the Data Recording Sheet.

Step 6   *Interpret Results.* The chart at the end of the lab illustrates Endurance Push-up Testing Norms for both males and females within each age category.

Modified Push-up (Females)

Step 1   *Starting Position.* The technique is modified for female subjects so that their knees are the first point of contact with the ground as opposed to the feet in the standard push-up position. This technique shortens the resistance arm which reduces the load placed upon the movement. The female subject begins by lying prone on the floor with the body extended. Have the subject place their hands approximately shoulders-width apart with the thumbs placed directly under the shoulders. The feet and knees should be together or no more than 6" apart. To help maintain rigid body position during the execution of the test, the subject can flex the knees to 90 degrees. This technique helps to reduce spinal hyperextension (sagging hips), which is often performed during push-ups from the knees. Have the subject lift the body to a point where the arms are completely extended. The legs should be in the bent-knee position with the body straight from the shoulders to the knees. A mat may be used to reduce the discomfort of knee contact with the ground.

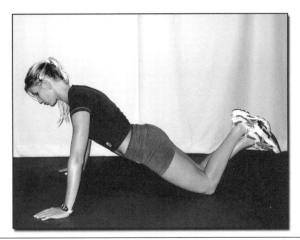 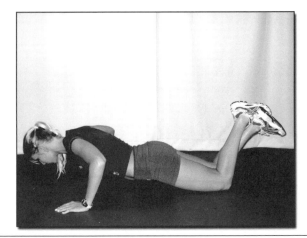

Step 2   *Begin Assessment.* Once the correct position is established the technician should give the "Go" command and begin timing. The subject should lower themselves in a rigid, straight position down to a point at which the elbows are at approximately 90° of flexion.

Step 3   *Movement Repetition.* The subject returns to the extended arm position by pushing upward until the elbows are fully extended. The subject may rest in the arm extended position, if necessary, during the assessment. This movement should be performed until volitional failure, technique breakdown, or the full duration of the test is completed. Count out loud each repetition the subject completes correctly.

Note: During the execution of the test be sure that the subject performs the movement through full ROM. It is common for a test subject to limit arm flexion and extension ROM to try and achieve a higher score. It is also important that the subject maintains rigid body position. At no time should the spine/torso be placed in a flexed or hyperextended position.

Common mechanical performance errors to look for include:

- Excessive scapular protraction and retraction without adequate elbow flexion
- Scapular elevation
- Excessive humeral abduction
- Hip flexion or hip and back extension from lack of core strength
- Incorrect wrist to elbow relationship
- Incorrect hand placement including inward rotation

Step 4   *Data Collection/Recording.* Record the number of repetitions successfully performed in one minute on the Data Recording Sheet.

Step 5   *Interpret Results.* The following chart illustrates Endurance Push-up Testing Norms for both males and females within each age category.

Push-up Test Recording Form

Name: _____   Date: _____

Gender: _____   Age: _____

Repetitions completed: _____   Fitness Rating: _____

Classifications for Push-up Test					
Men	**15-19 Y**	**20-29 Y**	**30-39 Y**	**40-49 Y**	**50-59 Y**	**60-69 Y**
Above Average	>28	>28	>21	>16	>12	>10
Average	22-28	21-28	17-21	13-16	10-12	8-10
Below Average	<22	<21	<17	<13	<10	<8
Women						
Above Average	>24	>20	>19	>14	>10	>8
Average	18-24	15-20	13-19	11-14	7-10	5-8
Below Average	<18	<15	<13	<11	<7	<5

Activity 6.8 Abdominal Curl-up Test

Activity Description

The muscles of the core and abdomen are predominately comprised of slow twitch muscle fibers. They are highly resistant to fatigue due to their constant responsibility in postural stabilization. The maintenance of adequate trunk strength and endurance are extremely important factors for healthy posture, the performance of general physical activity, and low back health. Many people are routinely affected by repetitive micro-trauma from poor movement biomechanics and improper posture caused by weakness, tightness, and imbalances of the trunk musculature.

Low back pain is the predominant cause for activity limitations in people under the age of 45. This phenomenon can be prevented with proper conditioning, specifically in the trunk musculature. Since the abdominals play such a large role in trunk health, it is very important to determine if there is adequate strength and endurance in this area. One way to assess the health of this region is with the abdominal curl-up test.

Historically, the sit-up was probably the most widely used muscle endurance test in fitness assessments. Recent literature has identified that the full sit-up is contraindicated due to the stress it places on the low back and that hip flexion accounts for 60 degrees of the traditional movement. Additionally, the hip flexors become increasingly involved when an individual's feet are held down by an outside force.

A recommended alternative to the full sit-up is an abdominal curl-up or crunch, which is defined as trunk flexion up to approximately 30 degrees. This type of half sit-up isolates the abdominal musculature better than any other type of sit-up studied. These facts have led to the use of the abdominal curl-up for better assessment of abdominal endurance. Numerous versions of the abdominal curl-up test have been developed over the last two decades as curl-up tests have become the dominant field test of muscular endurance in many fitness test batteries. Some of these tests include the Canadian partial curl-up, the Fit Youth Today (FYT) curl-up, the Modified trunk-curl, the Georgia Tech (GTCU) curl-up, and the Bench trunk-curl (BTC).

No matter which curl-up test is selected for an endurance assessment, it is how the test is administered that strongly influences the validity of the fitness test scores. When testing abdominal fitness, testers need to provide careful instructions on proper technique, conduct practice trials before the actual testing takes place, monitor technique and test protocols, and solicit maximum effort from subjects.

To reduce hip flexion and increase the ability of the test subject to control the movement pattern and speed, cadence tests have been developed. Advantages of curl-up tests using a cadence are seen in the fact that they emphasize controlled repetition rates, which reduce momentum forces and hip flexor innervation. This increases the validity of the test and eliminates potentially dangerous bouncing and ballistic actions in the hips and back. A disadvantage is that they are more difficult to administer to large groups, and subjects find various ways to modify their movements and still stay within the cadence.

The test for this lab experience is based upon endurance capabilities using a set pace. The test requires the subject to repetitively contract the abdominal musculature at a metronome paced 20 curl-ups per minute (40 beats · min^{-1}) for as many repetitions as possible up to 75. Each repetition should be performed slowly and controlled to the pace of the metronome. As soon as the subject cannot continue at the metronome pace, the test is stopped. Individuals that fail to reach at least the minimum requirements for adequate health in this area need to remedy the situation with appropriate exercises aimed at strengthening the region.

Some relevant concerns do exist when assessing trunk endurance. Some individuals suffer from low back problems, which can be aggravated with the movements used in this test. By properly screening applicants prior to testing, the test can be safely administered without injury. If an individual is classified as a potential risk, they should not be tested with this assessment procedure.

Activity Equipment

- Stop watch
- Gym mat
- Metronome

Procedures

The test requires a subject to perform a maximal number of repetitions at a set pace. Some individuals may reach failure early in the test. If this occurs, the test is stopped and the score is recorded. If an individual fails to perform the repetitions with a full range of motion or cannot maintain the 3 second per contraction pace they should stop the test. Incorrect movements should not be scored, this includes creating momentum from the floor to attain a mechanical advantage. If the subject fails to perform the movement correctly for more than three repetitions, they should be asked to stop the test.

Prior to testing, the subject should be instructed on proper movement technique. As in any test, he or she should meet the pre-test requirements of the test checklist. Following an adequate warm-up, the subject should perform the technique for a minimum of 3-4 repetitions to ensure that their ability and movement technique allow for safe testing protocols. If they cannot perform or are unable to follow the instructions listed below, he or she should not be tested.

Step 1   *Test Set Up.* Select an area with a solid flat surface. Do not perform the test on a flat bench. Make sure that the area selected is safe and the surrounding environment is appropriate for testing. Place a gym mat on the ground in an area that offers sufficient space for the assessment.

Step 2   *Starting Position.* Have the test subject assume the supine position with knees flexed and feet flat on the floor approximately 12" apart. The arms should be extended, palms resting on the thighs with fingertips pointing at the knees.

Step 3   *Begin Assessment.* Set the metronome for 40 beats · min⁻¹. On the "Go" command, the tester starts the metronome and the subject curls-up in a controlled manner until the fingers reach the top of the knees as the cadence sounds. Each beat represents a transitional change in the movement. The movements should be controlled and on pace with the metronome.

Step 4   *Movement Repetition.* The subject then returns to the starting position until the upper back makes contact with the mat while the abdominals remain contracted. This should be repeated until the subject cannot perform any more repetitions through the full ROM or the time expires.

Step 5   *Data Collection.* The technician should count out loud each correct repetition. If the subject performs 75 repetitions, stop the test and record the results. Subjects stopping before the terminal score of 75 repetitions should have their score recorded at the end of the test.

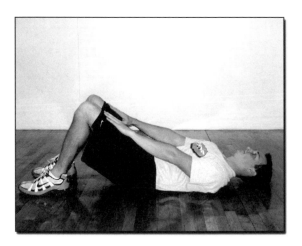 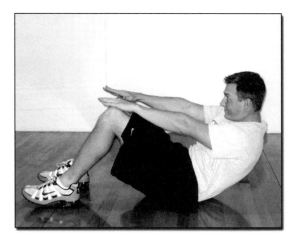

Step 6   *Interpretation of Results.* The table on the following page indicates the endurance ratings for trunk flexion for both males and females. It is based on the number of completed curl-ups for each age category. The table should be used to help interpret the test score.

Curl-up Test Recording Form

Name: _____   Date: _____

Gender: _____   Age: _____

Repetitions Completed: _____   Fitness Rating: _____

Classification for Abdominal Curl-up Test					
Men	**20-29 Y**	**30-39 Y**	**40-49 Y**	**50-59 Y**	**60-69 Y**
Above Average	≥21	≥18	≥18	≥17	≥16
Average	16-20	15-17	13-17	11-16	11-15
Below Average	<16	<15	<13	<11	<11
Women					
Above Average	≥20	≥19	≥19	≥19	≥17
Average	14-19	11-18	10-18	9-18	8-16
Below Average	<14	<11	<10	<9	<8

Lab Six Submission Form - Fitness Testing

1. Explain the anticipated blood pressure response (systolic and diastolic) during the performance of a submax VO_2 assessment.

   _____

   _____

   _____

2. Why is VO_2 adjusted for age?

   _____

   _____

3. What is the <u>non-adjusted</u> aerobic fitness level of a 185 pound, 45 year-old male subject with a 15 sec post test heart rate of 33 beats $\cdot$ min^{-1} (Forestry Step Test)?

   _____ ml $\cdot$ kg^{-1} $\cdot$ min^{-1}

4. What is the estimated VO_2max (age-adjusted) for the above sample client?

   _____ ml $\cdot$ kg^{-1} $\cdot$ min^{-1}

5. Using the information in the chart below, calculate the sample subject's VO_2max from the results of the One Mile Walk Test. Show all work and enter your results in the box.

Age	Weight	Gender	One Mile Walk time	10 sec. Post test HR	Estimated VO₂max ml • kg⁻¹ • min⁻¹
36	145	F	15:30	24	

   0.0769 x _____ lbs = _____ Value #1

   0.3877 x _____ years = _____ Value #2

   6.3150 x _____ gender = _____ Value #3

   3.2649 x _____ min. = _____ Value #4

   0.1565 x _____ HR = _____ Value #5

   132.853 – (_____ #1) – (_____ #2) + (_____ #3) – (_____ #4) – (_____ #5) = _____ ml $\cdot$ kg^{-1} $\cdot$ min^{-1}

Lab Six Submission Form - Fitness Testing

6. Name 4 reasons why men typically have a higher VO₂max than women.

    1. _____

    2. _____

    3. _____

    4. _____

7. A 35 year-old, 120 pound female, bench presses 55 pounds for 8 repetitions. What is her estimated 1RM bench press and what classification of strength does this person fall under according to the Relative Bench Press Norms? Show work.

    _____ Estimated 1RM   _____ Strength Classification

8. _____ is the predominant energy system used in multi-repetition strength tests.

9. Multi-repetition tests should attempt to reach muscle fatigue between _____ and _____ repetitions. Why?

    _____

    _____

10. What muscle group is innervated above 30° of trunk flexion during supine abdominal activities?

    _____

Lab Seven
Flexibility Assessment and Programming

Lab Seven corresponds to the following textbook reading:

Flexibility   Chapter 16

Lab Description

Flexibility is a primary component of health related fitness and is characterized by the ability or inability of a joint to move through a full range of motion (ROM). It is often the case that an individual will possess acceptable ROM capabilities in one joint or plane of motion and have poor ROM in another joint or movement plane. Many factors influence the ROM capabilities of an individual. They include, but are not limited to, aging, inactivity, muscle atrophy, muscle imbalances between agonist and antagonist groups, repetitive activities not performed through a full ROM or executed biomechanically incorrect, adhesions, loss of elasticity in connective tissue, as well as shortened tendons, fascia, and muscle fibers due to any of the previously listed. In addition, poor ROM capabilities are directly linked to physical ailments such as low back (repetitive) micro trauma, poor joint health, and reduced physical movement capabilities. Pain related limitations decrease activity, and therefore, reduce joint ROM. The upside to this is that the majority of the reasons used to explain why a person experiences limited ROM capabilities can be reversed through adherence to a well-designed flexibility program.

Lab seven introduces flexibility assessment and programming techniques that can be applied in different training situations. Personal trainers commonly utilize flexibility training techniques of varying nature in the exercise prescription for their clients. In order to properly prescribe and incorporate individualized flexibility protocols, you must first have full comprehension of the client's specific ROM needs. Needs analysis and determination start with physical assessments, visual observations, and client feedback. Incorporating a flexibility routine into a client's program without clear-cut objectives not only wastes the client's time, but may also result in negative outcomes. A well planned flexibility program based on a client's goals, ROM assessments, and biomechanical observations can have implications on program effectiveness and overall health.

Explored Procedures
- Flexibility assessment
- Flexibility training techniques
- Flexibility programming

Lab Objectives
- Understand the role of flexibility and the mechanics of the structures involved
- Successfully administer and interpret field flexibility assessments
- Identify and perform different flexibility training techniques for various body segments
- Identify contraindicated movements and applications that increase the risk for potential injury

Activity 7.1 Assessing Flexibility

Activity Description
The following section employs field flexibility assessments for different joint structures. The performance of the assessments can provide a trainer with valuable information pertaining to a client's ROM capabilities and needs. Many of the assessments can also serve as actual stretching techniques within a flexibility program.

The assessments serve to establish a baseline of flexibility and provide information about the client's movement capabilities and limitations. Arguably, the most valuable information pertaining to movement restrictions will occur during the actual observation of your client's performance of each activity. All training observations should be recorded in a detailed daily activity log for tracking purposes.

Procedures

Read through the six field flexibility assessments in Chapter 14 and then have your volunteer subject perform an adequate warm-up. Once the test subject is appropriately prepared, have the subject perform each assessment technique. Be sure to perform a bilateral assessment where applicable, as ROM differences between contralateral joints are common. Report your findings at the end of this section on the provided recording form below. Remember to be as detailed as possible when reporting your findings. **Note**: Instruct the subject to perform the movements in a controlled fashion and not to attempt to forcibly attain a position outside of his or her functional ROM.

Flexibility Assessment Recording Form

Name _____   Date _____

1. Shoulder Rotation   Assessed Structure _____

                                      Left Results _____   Right Results _____

Identify a stretch for the muscle group assessed _____

Identify a resistance training exercise that should be avoided if ROM is limited in the joint movement.

Exercise_____

2. Trunk Flexion   Assessed Structure _____

                                      Results _____

Identify a stretch for the muscle group assessed _____

Identify a resistance training exercise that should be avoided if ROM is limited in the joint movement.

Exercise_____

3. Trunk Extension   Assessed Structure _____

                                      Results _____

Identify a stretch for the muscle group assessed _____

Identify a resistance training exercise that should be avoided if ROM is limited in the joint movement.

Exercise_____

4. Hip Extension   Assessed Structure _____

                                  Left Results _____   Right Results _____

Identify a stretch for the muscle group assessed _____

Identify a resistance training exercise that should be avoided if ROM is limited in the joint movement.

Exercise_____

5. Knee Flexion   Assessed Structure _____

                                  Left Results _____   Right Results _____

Identify a stretch for the muscle group assessed _____

Identify a resistance training exercise that should be avoided if ROM is limited in the joint movement.

Exercise_____

6. Knee Extension   Assessed Structure _____

                                  Left Results _____   Right Results _____

Identify a stretch for the muscle group assessed _____

Identify a resistance training exercise that should be avoided if ROM is limited in the joint movement.

Exercise_____

Notes: This section is used to provide additional information pertaining to any findings. Due to the subjectivity of the evaluation, it is imperative that the tester (trainer) be as descriptive as possible when reporting problem areas.

Sample Trainer Notes:

John experienced acute pain and diminished ROM in left shoulder during the Apley Back Scratch Test. Upon further questioning, he indicated that he injured the left shoulder about 1 year ago and the pain comes and goes. I recommended Dr. Steve Burline to him for a more thorough analysis. It is important to avoid activity that causes pain in the shoulder until activity recommendations are made from Dr. Burline. Proceed as able.

Activity 7.2 Flexibility Training Techniques

Activity Description

The majority of flexibility training techniques employed by personal trainers will be directed at improving the elastic properties of intramuscular fascia. There are several flexibility training techniques that personal trainers should become proficient in to facilitate optimal results within their client's program. Chapter 16 contains descriptions and illustrations that can assist you in learning these flexibility training techniques and aid with the integration of these techniques into a comprehensive exercise program. It is important to note that many of the techniques employed by personal trainers require a level of professional skill and familiarity to ensure that the correct technique is adhered to and the prescription properly addresses the client's needs. Additionally, the flexibility program or techniques should be screened for client appropriateness to ensure that they do not have the potential to cause injury or harm to the client and that they attend to the specific needs and limitations of each client. There is a level of risk involved any time a trainer prescribes, implements, or performs flexibility training in a client's workout. The imposed risk can be greatly reduced by the trainer having a thorough understanding of the mechanics of the stretch, physical cues and communication, as well as identifying any contraindications to the performance of a particular exercise.

Static stretching is probably the most widely used flexibility training technique. It simply requires the user to assume a particular stretch position with the body segment/joint near or at full functional ROM and to hold the position for a predetermined period of time. Research indicates that for optimal results, the full ROM be held for 30-45 seconds, but logistics (discomfort tolerance, workout time constraints, program goals, etc.) may suggest a 15-20 second hold to be more realistic. Static stretching is favorable for clients that are beginning an exercise program and have limited experience with the physiological discomforts associated with more aggressive stretching techniques. Static stretching requires limited energy expenditure, may result in less muscle discomfort, and can assist in the reduction of muscular stress when performed following an adequate warm-up. Static stretching is ideally performed at the end of a workout when the tissue is at optimal temperature.

Procedure

The following static stretches are presented in Chapter 16 of your course textbook. Following the performance of an adequate warm-up, perform the designated movements and identify the soft tissue structures being stretched with each exercise. Each exercise should be held for a minimum of 15 seconds.

Example

Butterfly Stretch

Muscles involved: <u>Hip adductors</u>

Movement performed: <u>Hip abduction, partial hip external rotation</u>

<u>X</u> Performed

Supine Trunk Rotation

Muscles involved: _____

Movement performed: _____

_____ Performed

Seated Reach Trunk Rotator Stretch

Muscles involved: _____

Movement performed: _____

_____ Performed

Latissimus Dorsi Stretch from the Floor

Muscles involved: _____

Movement performed: _____

_____ Performed

Standing Adductor Stretch

Muscles involved: _____

Movement performed: _____

_____ Performed

Hip Flexor Stretch

Muscles involved: _____

Movement performed: _____

_____ Performed

Activity 7.3 Active-Assisted Stretching

Activity Description
Active-assisted stretching employs the use of an outside agent to attain full ROM. However, the outside agent (trainer or stationary object) may or may not increase the tension through the use of additional force application. The assistance can be used to attain greater movement range or serve a stable barrier in which the client is better able to maintain the stretched position to attain greater ROM. Similar to the static hold, the stretch should be sustained for approximately 30 seconds when employing active-assisted stretching exercises.

Procedures
Select a partner or test subject to perform the following flexibility activities and have them perform an adequate warm-up activity prior to performing the designated exercises. Following the warm-up, perform each activity. Upon completion of the activity, identify the structures that were involved in the exercise and document any observed limitations. In some cases, the flexibility technique will address a particular structure, whereas in others, more than one muscle group is being stretched. The stretches can be referenced in Chapter 16 of your course textbook.

Partner-Assisted Piriformis Stretch

Muscles involved: _____

Observed limitations: _____

_____ Performed

Partner-Assisted Quadricep Stretch

Muscles involved: _____

Observed limitations: _____

_____ Performed

Partner-Assisted Glute Stretch

Muscles involved: _____

Observed limitations: _____

_____ Performed

Partner-Assisted Gastrocnemius Stretch

Muscles involved: _____

Observed limitations: _____

_____ Performed

Activity 7.4 Dynamic Flexibility

Activity Description

Dynamic flexibility is a somewhat vague term in that it is not specific to a single functional application, nor is there a universally accepted definition for it. It basically encompasses movements that use a full range of motion throughout the performance of the exercise, independent of the movement speed. It does not necessarily denote the action as quick, slow, ballistic, or otherwise. It does though suggest that some percentage of the ROM limit is reached through the use of an isotonic contraction. Dynamic flexibility may be one of the most time-saving techniques available to the personal trainer because it can be used within safe limits of physical activity and allows for effective enhancement of flexibility while other training goals are being attained. Its efficacy is obvious when we look at what decreases flexibility in the aging population. Dynamic flexibility is used in conjunction with movement activities and therefore enables active bodies to maintain or increase ROM under conditions of elevated tissue temperature. Trainers do need to take caution in exercise selection so as not to place clients in compromising positions under load, especially when greater flexibility is necessary for the safe completion of the activity or exercise. Dynamic flexibility is useful, but like ballistic stretching, can become hazardous when used inappropriately or too aggressively. Ideally, dynamic flexibility uses controlled speeds to avoid activating a proprioceptive response that increases tension within the tissue.

Procedures

Review the following illustrations and descriptions to ascertain proper exercise technique for each dynamic flexibility activity. Once the information has been reviewed, perform a general warm-up. Following the warm-up, perform the movements using the illustrations and descriptions as a guide. Identify the muscles involved and the joint actions. In some cases, the dynamic flexibility techniques can serve as both flexibility and strengthening exercises, saving time while providing for efficient training response.

Lunge to High Knee

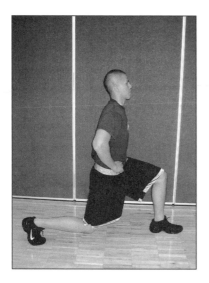
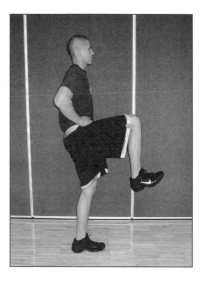

Standing in an upright posture with feet located under the hips, take a broad step backward, flexing both the front and back knee to the fullest range of motion. Once the hip has reached its greatest attainable range of motion, the back leg will be lifted forward and upward bringing the knee as high as possible toward the chest while balancing on the contralateral foot. Following the completion of the designated number of repetitions, the action should be switched to the other side.

Muscles being stretched: _____

Joint actions: _____

Wide Squat to Reach

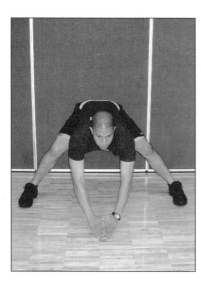
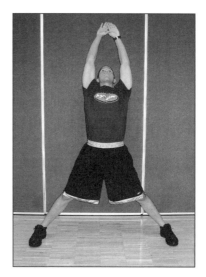

Starting with the widest attainable stance, reach both arms forward and downward while flexing the hip and knees. Once the fullest range of motion has been attained, the arms should be extended forward and upward as a standing posture is attained. The arms should attempt to reach above the body to the highest possible point.

Muscles being stretched: _____

Joint actions: _____

Alternating Toe Reach

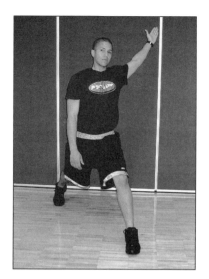 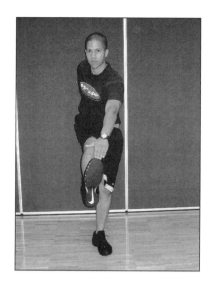

Standing in an upright position, step one leg backward while simultaneously reaching the contralateral arm upward and backward to a full range of motion. Once the fullest range of motion has been attained by both limbs, stabilize the body and move the limbs forward in the sagittal plane contacting the contralateral limbs at the furthest attainable point in front of the body. After completing the designated number of repetitions, switch to the other side.

Muscles being stretched: _____

Joint actions: _____

Scorpions

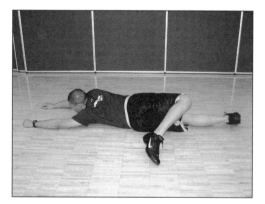 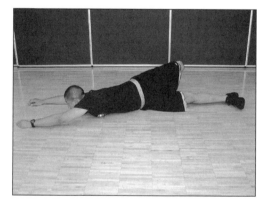

Lying in a prone position, reach one leg backward, upward, and across the body, flexing the knee so the toe makes contact with the floor. The arms should be extended forward against the ground and remain in that position during the activity. Once the leg has reached its fullest range of motion it should return to the start position as the contralateral leg follows the same movement across the body. Some trunk rotation will occur during the movement.

Muscles being stretched: _____

Joint actions: _____

Lateral Tucks to High Knee

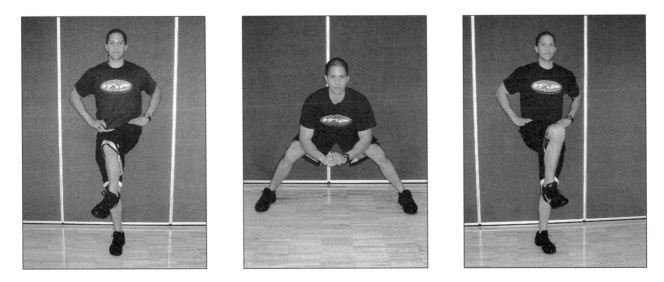

Standing in an upright posture with feet located under the hip, lift the step leg up to the highest attainable range of motion while bringing the knee toward the chest. Step laterally to the widest open leg stance and descend into a low tuck position, flexing both knees and hip to the fullest range of motion. Once the lowest point has been reached, stand upwards while drawing the contralateral leg toward the chest, establishing a balanced position. Repeat the movement back toward the start position tucking downward on each repetition.

Muscles being stretched: _____

Joint actions: _____

Opposite Heel Touch

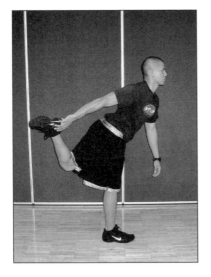 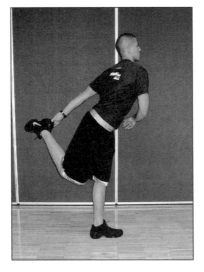

Standing in an upright posture with feet under the hips, lift one leg backward and medially upward while simultaneously reaching the contralateral arm back to touch the heel of the lifted foot. Stabilize at the fullest attainable range of motion before alternating to the other side.

Muscles being stretched: _____

Joint actions: _____

Activity 7.5 Proprioceptive Neuromuscular Facilitation (PNF)

Activity Description

Proprioceptive Neuromuscular Facilitation (PNF) describes more than simply the stretching of tissue. This ROM technique employs several neurophysiological mechanisms to synergistically facilitate new movement capabilities. PNF stretching is based upon inhibition, or reduced excitability of motor neurons in the antagonist musculature, and facilitation, or increased excitability of motor neurons in the agonist musculature. Together, the concurrent actions stimulate the CNS to create an optimal environment for tissue elongation, helping the muscle to attain a state of full range of motion. When this occurs, joint sensory endings, muscle spindles (proprioceptors that detect rate of change in length), and Golgi Tendon Organs (proprioceptors responsible for sensing change in tension) are activated, further affecting motor neuron excitability. In doing so, the muscle is able to reach ROM endpoints beyond that of the original position.

Essentially, the preceding paragraph suggests that we are able to trick the tissue into greater ROM capabilities. When a person actively moves his or her limb to a full ROM the body prevents it from further movement via proprioceptors, which dictate the tension and length response to prevent an overstretch injury. Once these structures determine an endpoint length and tension, range is limited. When a trainer holds the limb in that full ROM position, the client can then exert contractile force (isometric contraction) against the trainer's resistive force. In doing so, the proprioceptors assume a new environment of tension and readjust. This readjustment allows the limb to move beyond its previous terminal ROM. This contract/relax technique is often applied over three short (6-10 sec) periods per muscle group.

Procedures

Name: PNF Hamstring Stretch

Passive Stretch (Hold-Relax)

Step 1   The subject assumes a supine position on a mat. The trainer then passively stretches the subject's hamstring using the technique illustrated below.

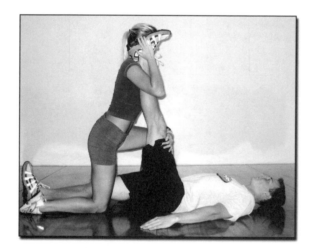

Step 2   The passive stretch is held for approximately 10 seconds.

Step 3   At the end of the 10 second hold, the trainer should instruct the subject to "push" the leg against the resistance provided by the trainer. The trainer should not allow the leg to move. This will produce an isometric contraction of the agonist muscle group. The isometric contraction should last for approximately 4 to 6 seconds.

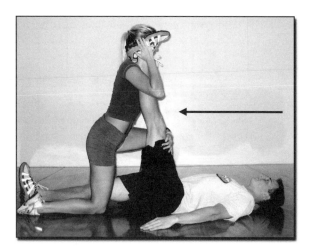

Step 4   Following the contraction, the limb should be re-stretched to a new attainable position.

Step 5   Repeat steps 2-4. The passive stretch between each isometric contraction should last approximately 10 seconds. The subject can slightly increase the intensity of the isometric contraction on each succeeding trial. Repeat the procedure 3 times.

Name: PNF Hamstring Stretch

Active Stretch (Contract-Relax)

Step 1   The subject assumes a supine position on a mat. The trainer then passively stretches the subject's hamstring using the technique illustrated below.

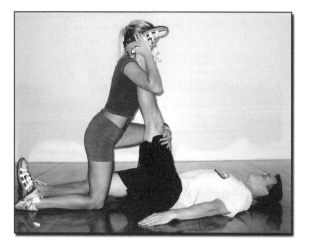

Step 2   Hold the position for 6-10 seconds.

Step 3   At the end of the isometric hold duration, the trainer instructs the subject to actively "pull" the leg backward by flexing the hip and quadricep. The activation of the subject's hip flexor group will temporarily increase the ROM of the hamstring group. This pull phase should last for approximately 4 to 6 seconds.

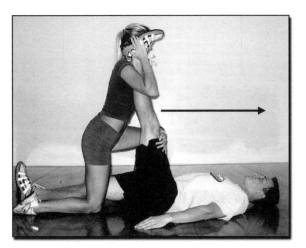

Step 4   At the end of the contraction phase, the subject should relax the hip flexor group and the trainer will then passively stretch the hamstring, holding the end range of motion for 10 seconds.

Step 5   Repeat Steps 2-4 up to 3 times.

Activity 7.6 Creating a Flexibility Circuit

Activity Description
Prescribing flexibility activities in a personal training session can be done in a variety of ways. Dynamic flexibility techniques can be programmed as part of a comprehensive warm-up or utilized within the training session. Static stretching techniques can be used as part of the cooldown activities or can be integrated within the exercise program. Flexibility circuits can also be used as a designated segment of the exercise program at anytime, consistent with specific goal attainment.

Procedures
Create a flexibility circuit using any of the flexibility program techniques outlined in your course text. Activities may be dynamic, static, or a combination of the two. Complete the chart by identifying the stretch activity and the type or mode of flexibility. Also, include the recommended duration for the stretch, or repetitions performed, if the activity is dynamic or PNF.

	Stretch	Mode of Flexibility	Time or repetitions
Example: **Shoulder Flexors**	**Shoulder Flexor Stretch**	**Static**	**15 sec**
Trunk Rotators			
Trunk Extensors			
Shoulder Extensors			
Hip Adductors			
Hip Extensors			
Hip Flexors			
Plantar Flexors			

Lab Seven Submission Form – Flexibility Assessment and Programming

1. What is the difference between dynamic stretching and active stretching?

_____

2. What is the optimal length of time you should hold a static stretch? _____ seconds

3. What physiological benefits are derived from the performance of a warm–up before performing a flexibility exercise?

_____

_____

_____

4. Your client is found to have poor ROM in the latissimus dorsi muscle group. Answer the following questions pertaining to this condition.

    A. List two resistance training exercises that may be difficult to perform properly.

        _____

        _____

    B. List two stretches that should be included in the program to increase range of motion in the muscle group.

        _____

        _____

5. Your client is found to have poor ROM in the hamstring muscle group. Answer the following questions pertaining to this condition.

    A. List two resistance training exercises that may be difficult to perform properly.

        _____

        _____

    B. List two stretches that should be included in the program to increase range of motion in the muscle group.

        _____

        _____

6. What resistance training exercise could be employed to dynamically stretch the hip flexor?

_____

7. Why does the knee have to be in the extended position to stretch the gastrocnemius?

_____

_____

8. What specific muscle is being stretched during the active hip flexor stretch?

_____

9. True or False. Performance of the seated back flexion stretch is designed to increase the length of the parallel

   running, spinal ligamentous structures. _____

10. If your new client has poor range of motion when attempting shoulder flexion, which exercise listed below would
    your client have difficulty performing and should be avoided until better ROM capabilities are achieved?

Bench Press	Yes	No
Overhead Press (military)	Yes	No
Dumbbell Lateral Raises	Yes	No

Lab Eight
Aerobic Exercise Prescription, Caloric Expenditure, and MET Intensity

Lab Eight corresponds to the following textbook reading:

Programming for Cardiovascular Fitness   Chapter 17

Lab Description

The term "aerobic" refers to the presence of oxygen in energy metabolism. Oxygen is a key component in the reactions needed to satisfy the energy demands of prolonged activity or exercise and constitutes the primary gas for cellular respiration. The link between aerobic exercise and caloric expenditure comes from the process of producing cellular energy with oxygen for continuous work. Oxidative phosphorylation is the term used to describe the chain of events that allows oxygen to provide the body with energy.

During all physical states, the body requires oxygen to carry on normal biological function. At rest, the oxygen demands of the body are relatively low, satisfying only the basic requirements of cellular activity. Each person's relative demand will vary based on factors like size and fitness level. The specific amount of oxygen used at rest can be quantified by a measurement of oxygen known as a MET, or metabolic equivalent of resting oxygen uptake. It represents an oxygen value of 3.5 ml· kg^{-1}· min^{-1}. As you can see from the measurement unit, the way it becomes relative to an individual is by the weight of that person in kilograms. When the body moves from a resting state to an active state the oxygen demands increase. MET intensity is used to quantify the relative amount of oxygen needed to perform the task at any intensity level. Exercise intensity and MET values increase linearly indicating that the harder the body works the more oxygen it requires. This yields positive effects on weight management due to the fact that for every liter of oxygen used by the body it will burn approximately 5 calories, depending on the specific fuel source.

From an overall needs analysis, the maintenance/improvement of cardiorespiratory endurance/function (VO_2) should be considered the most important component to health related fitness. The activities employed that engage the cardiorespiratory system have positive effects on the other four components of fitness. Regular aerobic exercise translates into reduced risk for disease, better physical functionality, and improved quality of life. Having a thorough understanding of the physiological mechanisms of cardiovascular function and the adaptation response of the body to cardiovascular endurance training is necessary to prescribe safe and effective exercise.

The following activities will explore the physiological adaptations to exercise, various methods of developing an aerobic exercise prescription, the link between aerobic activity and caloric expenditure, and how to calculate the caloric intensity of an activity based on the amount of oxygen consumed (MET Intensity).

Explored Procedures

- Use of the Max Heart Rate Formula and Method for cardiovascular exercise prescription
- Use of the Heart Rate Reserve and Karvonen Formula for cardiovascular exercise prescription
- Use of the RPE scale for the monitoring of cardiovascular exercise intensity
- Calculation of caloric expenditure based on exercise intensity and oxygen utilization
- Development of cardiorespiratory training programs using multi-modalities

Lab Objectives

- Understand the physiological adaptations to aerobic exercise
- Identify appropriate modes of cardiovascular exercise based on a client's goals, interests, and abilities
- Identify appropriate starting points for intensity and duration based on quantified individual parameters
- Understand the relationship between oxygen utilization and caloric expenditure
- Successfully prescribe aerobic exercise intensities based on individual findings

Physiological Adaptations to Aerobic Exercise

As you now know, understanding the physiological adaptations to aerobic exercise is a fundamental component in the development of a proper exercise prescription. The specific prescription for a client will come from a needs analysis based on evaluative criteria.

Research has found that aerobic training can increase aerobic capacity (VO_2) by up to 15%-30% with consistent aerobic conditioning. This value may increase even more with continued training at progressively higher intensities. The specific physiological adaptations that occur in response to regular aerobic training include: enhanced aerobic enzyme activity, which facilitates more efficient carbohydrate and lipid breakdown; increased muscle fiber capillary density, which allows for increased oxygen to the working muscles and increased by-product waste removal; and increased mitochondrial density, contributing to greater oxygen utilization. At the same time, the heart responds by increasing contractile force and stroke volume which in turn decreases the resting and exercise heart rate response at the same relative intensities. Together, cardiac and skeletal muscle adaptations increase the body's capacity to circulate, deliver, and utilize oxygen, which translates to increases in VO_2 max and a more efficient cardiorespiratory system.

Aerobic Training Intensities

The term "Training Intensity" refers to the amount of physical exertion the body experiences when performing an activity or exercise. In the case of aerobic exercise, the intensity reflects the speed of the movement, or resistance to the movement, and is usually physiologically quantified by the subject's heart rate response at a given workload. For maximal gains in cardiorespiratory fitness to take place, ideal training intensity zones have been established which utilize specific heart rate responses based on workloads. The two most commonly accepted methods of calculating training intensity zones are based on heart rate and utilize either the Heart Rate Max Formula or Heart Rate Reserve Formula (HRR). The formulas use a predicted maximum heart rate based on age. Based on bell curve theory, the formulas may be off as much as 10-24 beats $\cdot$ min^{-1} in 32% of the population (SD=10-12 bpm). For this reason, RPE should be used in conjunction with HRmax predictions to improve the accuracy of the prescribed training zones.

RPE stands for rate of perceived exertion. It quantifies intensity or exertion levels using the Borg Scale - Rate of Perceived Exertion. The scale uses a 1-10 or 6-20 rating in which exercisers verbally communicate their level of intensity by looking at the scale and providing the number that corresponds with their perceived exertion. The Borg Scale can help reduce estimation errors in predicted training zones by comparing the relative intensity to the physical exertion perceived by the exerciser. For example, if a person is thought to be training at 75% of their HRmax and only experiencing a 10 on the 20-point scale they are likely not at the desired intensity and therefore not maximizing training results. Personal trainers can effectively use the Borg Scale to make the predictive formulas more accurate. Modifications should be made to adjust the heart rate zone to the level required for goal specific training adaptations.

The following lab activity outlines how to calculate aerobic training intensities for maximal gains in cardiorespiratory fitness. It is important to note that the percent-range (heart rate) calculations used for the Max Heart Rate Method and Heart Rate Reserve Formula are for maximal gains in CRF and may be too intense for many beginner exercisers, particularly deconditioned participants.

Activity 8.1 Calculating Maximum Heart Rate and Aerobic Training Intensities

Activity Description

After selecting the mode(s) of cardiovascular training that will be incorporated into a client's exercise prescription, the trainer must establish the appropriate intensity for the training. To do this, one must first identify the client's maximum heart rate. If a maximal test is not used to determine the actual maximum heart rate, then the heart rate value can be predicted using an indirect method. Once the heart rate max has been determined, the trainer can use this information to compute an appropriate training intensity using one of several methods: Max Heart Rate, Heart Rate Reserve, and/ or RPE.

Procedures

This activity requires the calculation of a subject's training intensities using two different methods (you have the option of calculating your own). Once the target heart rate zone (THRZ) has been established, you will have the subject exercise until a steady-state HR within the zone is reached. RPE will then be used to validate the calculations. Be sure to read through the entire lab activity prior to performing the procedures.

Step 1   Assess the resting heart rate and record base information:

Resting Heart Rate of subject _____ beats • min^{-1}

Age of subject _____

Mode of cardiorespiratory activity selected _____

Step 2   Calculate Maximum Heart Rate for your subject using the Indirect Method.

220 – Age = predicted Max Heart Rate

220 – _____ subject's age = _____ predicted Max Heart Rate

Record subject's predicted Max Heart Rate value _____ beats • min^{-1}

Step 3   Calculate subject's Target Heart Rate Zone using Max Heart Rate Method and the recommended (75%-90%) training intensities.

Sample Subject: 45 year-old male with a resting heart rate of 77 beats • min^{-1}

Find the predicted max heart rate.

220 – **45** = 175 beats • min^{-1}

Find the recommended training zones using the Max Heart Rate Method and corresponding intensity ranges.

175 beats • min^{-1} x **.75** = 130 beats • min^{-1} (Low-end)
175 beats • min^{-1} x **.90** = 158 beats • min^{-1} (High-end)

Target Heart Rate Zone = 130 beats • min^{-1} to 158 beats • min^{-1}

Enter the predicted max heart rate of the subject from Step 2 and calculate the Target Heart Zone using the intensities provided.

_____ Max HR x (.75) = _____ (L)

_____ Max HR x (.90) = _____ (H)

Record the low end and high end of the training zone.

Target Heart Rate Zone = (L) _____ to (H) _____ beats • min^{-1}

Step 4   Calculate subject's Target Heart Rate Zone using the Heart Rate Reserve (HRR) method and recommended corresponding training intensities (60%-80%) for use with the Karvonen Formula.

Karvonen Formula/Heart Rate Reserve Method

Max HR – Resting HR (RHR) = Heart Rate Reserve (HRR)
{HRR x (training intensity)} + RHR = Target Heart Rate

Sample Subject: 45 year-old male with a resting heart rate of 77 beats $\cdot$ min^{-1}

Find the Max Heart Rate.

220 – **45** = 175 beats $\cdot$ min^{-1}

Find recommended training zones using HRR method and corresponding intensity ranges.

Max Heart Rate – Resting Heart Rate = Heart Rate Reserve

175 beats $\cdot$ min^{-1} – **77** beats $\cdot$ min^{-1} = 98 beats $\cdot$ min^{-1}

Heart Rate Reserve = 98 beats $\cdot$ min^{-1}

(Heart Rate Reserve x Training Intensity) + Resting Heart Rate = Target Heart Rate

Low-end   98 beats $\cdot$ min^{-1} x **.60** = 58 + 77 beats $\cdot$ min^{-1} = 135 beats $\cdot$ min^{-1}

High-end   98 beats $\cdot$ min^{-1} x **.80** = 78 + 77 beats $\cdot$ min^{-1} = 155 beats $\cdot$ min^{-1}

HRR Target Training Zones = 135 beats $\cdot$ min^{-1} to 155 beats $\cdot$ min^{-1}

Enter the predicted max heart rate and resting heart rate of the subject from Step 2 and calculate the Target Heart Rate Zone using the intensities provided.

Max HR – Resting HR = Heart Rate Reserve

_____ Max HR – _____ Resting Heart Rate = _____ Heart Rate Reserve

Record Value _____

_____ Heart Rate Reserve x (.60) + _____ Resting Heart Rate = _____ Target Heart Rate Zone (L)

Record Value _____ THRZ (L)

_____ Heart Rate Reserve x (.80) + _____ Resting Heart Rate = _____ Target Heart Rate Zone (H)

Record Value _____ THRZ (H)

Target Heart Rate Zone = (L) _____ to (H) _____ beats $\cdot$ min^{-1}

Step 5   Have the test subject begin exercise using the mode selected, gradually increasing the intensity until the desired level is reached (75% of predicted HRmax or 60% of the HRR Formula). Incorporate the use of the Rating of Perceived Exertion Scale. Ask the subject how they feel at the given workload. A 12-14 Rating on the 6 to 20 scale correlates to the recommended 60% to 80% HRR method and 75% to 90% HRmax method. If they are below or above the 12 value adjust the speed, resistance, or incline until the subject feels the exertion is beyond light. For most people this does not require much work. Record the heart rate when they have reached a steady-state heart rate in the designated zone. Do the same for the high end of the range (90% of predicted HRmax or 80% of the HRR Formula) reaching a RPE value of 14 or just above somewhat hard. Use all the data to ascertain the closest heart rate equivalent.

Step 6   Record the adjusted target heart rate zone _____ to _____ beats • min^{-1}

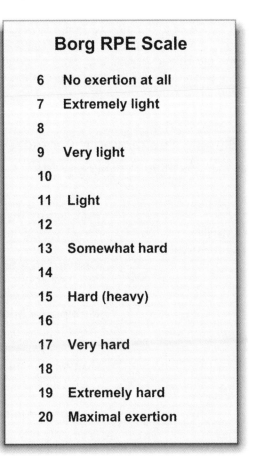

Activity 8.2 Converting METs to Kcals

Activity Description
The textbook explains how energy expenditure can be expressed in several different ways. The five most common expressions of energy include:

- VO_2 (L • min^{-1})
- VO_2 (ml • kg^{-1} • min^{-1})
- METs
- Kcal • min^{-1}
- Kcal • kg^{-1} • hr^{-1}

It should be noted that the expression either reflects a measure of oxygen or calories. For every liter of oxygen used by the body, there is a caloric value associated with it. The exact caloric expenditure is dependent on the energy used to fuel the metabolic requirements of the body (i.e., breakdown of fat, protein, or carbohydrates). This is expressed as the Respiratory Quotient (RQ). The RQ is used to separate the inherent differences in the chemical composition of carbohydrates, lipids, and proteins. Different amounts of oxygen are needed to oxidize carbon and hydrogen atoms to carbon dioxide and water. The RQ value for carbohydrates is 1.0 providing the most efficient energy. The RQ value for lipids is .7, while protein is .82. A mixed use of energy is valued at .825. There is a net caloric expenditure of 5, 4.7, and 4.8 Kcal • L^{-1} for carbohydrates, fat, and protein, respectively. Since it cannot be determined how the energy is being derived without calculating the subject's Respiratory Exchange Ratio (R), the value of 5 Kcal • L^{-1} of oxygen has been universally accepted as the caloric equivalent for oxygen utilization.

Identifying the oxygen demand of an activity allows the activity to reflect a caloric requirement. The two main components for calculating the caloric cost of an activity are recognizing that for every liter of O_2 used approximately 5 calories are expended and that 1 MET is equal to 3.5 ml $\bullet$ kg^{-1} $\bullet$ min^{-1}. Scientists have been able to assign a MET intensity to most activities by measuring the oxygen used during their performance. Once the MET value of the activity is known for a given intensity, the caloric expenditure can be derived by factoring in the weight of the individual and the duration of time it is performed. This is the same method used by cardiovascular equipment to identify the calories expended when using the machine.

Sample Conversion References
220 lb. man, 30 minutes using a 10 MET Activity

Calculating METs from VO₂
VO_2 = 35 ml $\bullet$ kg^{-1} $\bullet$ min^{-1}
Divide VO_2 by 3.5 ml $\bullet$ kg^{-1} $\bullet$ min^{-1} (1 MET)
35 ml $\bullet$ kg^{-1} $\bullet$ min^{-1} $\div$ 3.5 ml $\bullet$ kg^{-1} $\bullet$ min^{-1} = 10 METs

Convert ml to L (1 ml = .001 L)
1 ml = .001 L
35 ml = .035 L

Convert pounds to kilograms
1 lb = 2.2 kg
220 lb = 100 kg

Convert liters of O₂ to calories
1 L of O_2 = 5 kcal
10 L x 5 kcal = 50 kcal

Calculating calories from METs
Convert METs to VO_2
10 METs = 35 ml $\bullet$ kg^{-1} $\bullet$ min^{-1}

Convert VO₂ to liters of O₂ (1L = 1000 ml)
35 ml $\bullet$ kg^{-1} $\bullet$ min^{-1} = .035 L $\bullet$ kg^{-1} $\bullet$ min^{-1}

Multiply by kilograms of body weight
.035 L $\bullet$ kg^{-1} $\bullet$ min^{-1} x 100 kg = 3.5 L $\bullet$ min^{-1}

Convert L $\bullet$ min^{-1} to calories
3.5 L $\bullet$ min^{-1} x 5 kcal = 17.5 kcal $\bullet$ min^{-1}

Multiply by minutes of activity
17.5 kcal $\bullet$ min^{-1} x 30 minutes = 525 kcal total expenditure

Procedures
At rest the body uses 3.5 ml $\bullet$ kg^{-1} $\bullet$ min^{-1} or 1 MET. The following example demonstrates the conversion of METs into calories at rest. The value only accounts for the oxygen requirement of inactive tissue. It does not reflect eating, digestion, moving, or any other daily requirements that are calculated for daily need. After reviewing the formula, calculate your own metabolic rate using the MET energy conversion equation.

Calculate the caloric expenditure of a 155-pound person at rest.

1 MET = 3.5 ml $\bullet$ kg^{-1} $\bullet$ min^{-1}

155 lbs $\div$ 2.2 = 70.5 kg

70.5 kg x 3.5 ml $\bullet$ kg^{-1} $\bullet$ min^{-1} = 246.75 ml $\bullet$ min^{-1}

246.75 ml $\bullet$ min^{-1} x .001 L/ml = 0.24675 L $\bullet$ min^{-1}

0.24675 L $\bullet$ min^{-1} x 5 Kcal $\bullet$ L^{-1} = 1.23375 kcal $\bullet$ min^{-1}

1.23375 kcal $\bullet$ min^{-1} x 60 min $\bullet$ hour^{-1} = 74 kcal $\bullet$ hour^{-1}

74 kcal $\bullet$ hour^{-1} x 24 hours $\bullet$ day^{-1} = 1776 kcal $\bullet$ day^{-1}

In the spaces provided, calculate your personal caloric expenditure at rest.

Activity oxygen requirement = 1 MET or 3.5 ml $\bullet$ kg^{-1} $\bullet$ min^{-1}

Step 1   Divide your bodyweight in pounds by 2.2 to get bodyweight in kilograms

_____ lbs. ÷ 2.2 = _____ kg

Step 2   Multiply bodyweight in kilograms by 1 MET to get milliliters of oxygen used per minute

_____ kg x 3.5 ml $\bullet$ kg^{-1} $\bullet$ min^{-1} = _____ ml $\bullet$ min^{-1}

Step 3   Convert milliliters of oxygen per minute to liters of oxygen per minute

_____ ml $\bullet$ min^{-1} x .001 = _____ L $\bullet$ min^{-1}

Step 4   Multiply liters of oxygen by 5 calories per liter to get calories expended per minute

_____ L $\bullet$ min^{-1} x 5 kcal $\bullet$ L^{-1} = _____ kcal $\bullet$ min^{-1}

Step 5   Multiply calories per minute by the minutes in an hour to get calories expended per hour

_____ kcal $\bullet$ min^{-1} x 60 min $\bullet$ hour^{-1} = _____ kcal $\bullet$ hour^{-1}

Step 6   Multiply calories per hour by 24 hours to get calories expended per day

_____ kcal $\bullet$ hour^{-1} x 24 hours $\bullet$ day^{-1} = _____ kcal $\bullet$ day^{-1}

Activity 8.3 Practical Application of METs Case Study

Activity Description
As a person goes from a resting state to an active state the metabolic demands increase. The exact metabolic increase is dependent upon the activity done and the intensity in which it is performed. Using the information that you have learned about oxygen utilization and the relationship it has to caloric expenditure, read through the following case study and perform all designated caloric conversions. This case study will provide you with a better understanding of how to convert the MET intensity of an activity into caloric expenditure, as well as provide you with a better understanding of the relevance of this knowledge.

Procedures
Your client is a 148-pound female who wants to lose body fat. She is training three times per week under your supervision and, at your instruction, has been attempting to expend a minimum of 200 calories per day through sustained physical activity. During a Monday training session, she reports that the only sustained physical activity she was able to do over the weekend was 30 minutes of lawn raking. Does this qualify as continuous physical activity and meet your recommendation of a 200-calorie expenditure?

Step 1   Find out the MET intensity for the activity in the MET intensity appendix in the back of the lab manual.

Record MET intensity _____

Step 2   Convert MET intensity to absolute oxygen utilization represented as $ml \cdot kg^{-1} \cdot min^{-1}$.

$$\underline{\hspace{2cm}} \text{ METS x } 3.5 \text{ } ml \cdot kg^{-1} \cdot min^{-1} = \underline{\hspace{2cm}} \text{ } ml \cdot kg^{-1} \cdot min^{-1}$$

Step 3   Convert absolute oxygen utilization to relative oxygen utilization by multiplying the subject's weight in kilograms by the absolute oxygen utilization value from Step 2. Remember to first divide her weight in pounds by 2.2 to convert to kilograms.

$$\underline{\hspace{2cm}} \text{ kg x } \underline{\hspace{2cm}} \text{ } ml \cdot kg^{-1} \cdot min^{-1} = \underline{\hspace{2cm}} \text{ } ml \cdot min^{-1}$$

Step 4   Convert $ml \cdot min^{-1}$ to $L \cdot min^{-1}$ by multiplying by .001.

$$\underline{\hspace{2cm}} \text{ } ml \cdot min^{-1} \text{ x } .001 = \underline{\hspace{2cm}} \text{ } L \cdot min^{-1}$$

Step 5   Convert the oxygen used in $L \cdot min^{-1}$ from Step 4 to $kcal \cdot min^{-1}$ by multiplying the values from Step 4 by 5 kcals.

$$\underline{\hspace{2cm}} \text{ } L \cdot min^{-1} \text{ x } 5 \text{ } kcal \cdot L^{-1} = \underline{\hspace{2cm}} \text{ } kcal \cdot min^{-1}$$

Step 6   Multiply $kcal \cdot min^{-1}$ by total number of minutes she reports for the activity.

$$\underline{\hspace{2cm}} \text{ } kcal \cdot min^{-1} \text{ x } \underline{\hspace{2cm}} \text{ } min = \underline{\hspace{2cm}} kcal \text{ expended}$$

Does this value meet your recommendations?   Y or N

Activity 8.4 Establishing Training Zones Based on MET Intensity

Procedures

Cardiovascular training zones can also be based on MET intensities. The recommended training zones used for VO_2max is 60%-80%. Using the predicted VO_2max from Lab Six, calculate the subject's MET intensity training zones from the results of the submax VO_2 assessment.

Step 1   Record the VO_2max from one of the cardiovascular activities performed in Lab Six.

Predicted (VO_2max) $\underline{\hspace{2cm}}$ $ml \cdot kg^{-1} \cdot min^{-1}$

Step 2   Divide the VO_2max by 1 MET.

$VO_2max \div 3.5 \text{ } ml \cdot kg^{-1} \cdot min^{-1} = \underline{\hspace{2cm}}$ Max MET Value

Record Max MET Value $\underline{\hspace{2cm}}$

Step 3   Calculate the MET Training Zone using 60%-80% intensity.

Max MET Value $\underline{\hspace{2cm}}$ x 60% = $\underline{\hspace{2cm}}$

Max MET Value $\underline{\hspace{2cm}}$ x 80% = $\underline{\hspace{2cm}}$

MET Training Zone = $\underline{\hspace{2cm}}$ to $\underline{\hspace{2cm}}$

Step 4   Providing MET Intensity Training Zones means very little for practical implementation and tracking. Therefore, the MET intensities must be converted into Target Heart Rate Zones. Determine the Heart Rate that reflects the MET Training Zone by identifying the steady-state heart rates that occur when exercising at the defined MET intensity. On a cardiovascular machine that provides METs, have the subject exercise at the 60% MET training zone value until steady-state heart rate is attained and record the heart rate value. Increase the MET level to the 80% MET training zone and have the subject exercise until steady-state heart rate is again reached and record the heart rate value.

60% MET Zone _____ beats • min^{-1}

80% MET Zone _____ beats • min^{-1}

Target Heart Rate Zone _____ beats • min^{-1} to _____ beats • min^{-1}

Step 5   Using the MET Intensity Appendix in the back of the lab book, find activities with similar MET intensities to recommend quantifiable daily caloric expenditure options.

Establishing training zones based on VO$_2$max may be more reliable due to the potential errors involved with estimating an individual's maximum heart rate through the use of the indirect formula. However, this method is not without error when using a predicted VO$_2$max from a submax test.

Note: Leaning on the machine or not adhering to proper exercise form will lead to inaccurate training zones and usually result in less caloric expenditure.

Activity 8.5 Creating a Cardiovascular Circuit

Activity Description

Weight loss is probably the most common goal of most personal training clients and can be addressed in a variety of ways. No matter what method is selected, the same premise must apply "To reduce body fat one must burn calories or reduce consumption of calories to create a negative caloric balance." It makes sense that the focus of the training should be directed at caloric expenditure. This concept of caloric expenditure explains why aerobic training is commonly employed for this goal. Aerobic activity is constant and continuous, and it requires more energy expenditure than traditional weight training for the same duration because of the rest intervals used for resistance training activities. Additionally, the energy system that supplies the body with the most fuel for a moderately intense, continuous activity preys on adipose tissue. However, the need for resistance training cannot be neglected as elevations in RMR and the maintenance of muscle mass contribute to greater caloric expenditure. Additionally, aerobic training with concurrent caloric restriction often causes the loss of lean mass which negatively affects body composition.

The use of cross training and circuits are ideal for weight loss because they can utilize many different modes of training applied as continuous activity. The average resistance training session lasting one hour has about 20 minutes of actual training with forty minutes of rest. For this reason, weight training does not burn many calories per hour. When weight training is combined with aerobic training, the result is multiple muscle group and energy system activation. You get the benefits of resistance training, incorporate more muscle tissue than used in aerobic training alone, avoid excessive fatigue in any particular muscle group, maintain better focus and reduce boredom, burn more calories, provide different activities, and reach more components of fitness than cardiovascular or strength training can independently. It also allows for innovative and creative ideas for goal attainment and training enjoyment.

The following represents a sample where the THRZ is above 70% HRmax for 45-60 minutes and rest only occurs during station transitions, hydration, or if needed for safety purposes.

Station 1: Bike	3 min
Station 2: Jump rope	1.5 min
Station 3: Internal/external rotation	15 reps
Station 4: Body squats	30 reps
Station 5: Physioball push-ups	12 reps or as able
Station 6: Modified pull-ups	10-15 reps
Station 7: Jump rope	1 min
Station 8: Single leg squats	10 reps per side
Station 9: Medicine ball torso twists	20 reps
Station 10: Supine physioball leg curls	15 reps
Station 12: Medicine ball chest pass	20 reps
Station 13: 15" Box stepping	1.5 min
Station 14: High row with therabands	25 reps
Station 15: Trunk flexion	12 reps

This can be performed twice in an hour with significant caloric expenditure. The energy will come from multiple systems if the heart rate is maintained and transitions are of short duration. A heart rate monitor can be used to keep the rate between established training zone values.

Procedures

You have a 42 year-old, female client. She has been working with you for one year and has made great improvements in strength and endurance. She performs cardiovascular exercise three days per week, but really does not enjoy it and has low motivation to train at higher intensities. She likes to lift weights and is interested in further reducing her body fat without really doing much more aerobic training. She wants to know how she can use weight training to burn more calories. Construct a one-day training circuit to increase her caloric expenditure while emphasizing resistance training. You have dumbbells, a medicine ball, an aerobic step, and a stationary bike at your disposal. Use the corresponding table for your exercise prescription.

Note: Resistance training activities and techniques are covered in Chapter 19 of the course textbook.

MET Intensity Goal   _____ METs

Target Heart Rate Zone   _____ beats • min^{-1}

Time/Duration   _____ minutes

Calories Burned   _____ kcal

Day 1 Exercises	Reps or Time
1.	
2.	
3.	
4.	
5.	
6.	
7.	
8.	
9.	
10.	
11.	
12.	
13.	

Lab Eight Submission Form - Aerobic Exercise Prescription, Caloric Expenditure, and MET Intensity

1. To lower the risk of developing cardiovascular disease, the established minimum recommendation for sustained physical activity per day is _____ minutes, or _____ kcal to _____ kcal expenditure.

2. Aerobic training can increase aerobic capacity (VO_2) by _____% to _____% from consistent aerobic conditioning.

3. List 4 physiological adaptations to cardiovascular training that contribute to improved cardiorespiratory fitness.

   A. _____

   B. _____

   C. _____

   D. _____

4. A training intensity of ____% to ____% VO_2max is ideal for healthy individuals training for improved cardiorespiratory fitness.

5. As part of the exercise prescription for your new client, you incorporate ten minutes of cardiovascular exercise. They are overweight and extremely deconditioned. How would you choose the level of intensity for the mode of cardiovascular exercise prescribed? Include heart rate response and any other quantifiable measures in your explanation.

   _____

   _____

   _____

   _____

6. Your new client is a 32 year-old male with a resting heart rate of 75. In the space below, calculate his target heart rate for a 75% training intensity using the HRR method. Show all work.

   _____ beats • min^{-1}

Lab Eight Submission Form - Aerobic Exercise Prescription, Caloric Expenditure, and MET Intensity

7. What effect does leaning on the stair climber have on caloric expenditure and how does this affect the calories calculated by the machine?

    _____

    _____

8. Your client has been biking for 15 minutes and, according to your calculations, has maintained steady-state heart rate of 80% max heart rate for 12 minutes. When asked how she feels according to the original Borg Rating Scale she reports a 10 on the 20 point scale. What does this mean? Does her program need modification?

    _____

    _____

    _____

    _____

    _____

9. A VO_2max of 35 ml $\bullet$ kg $\bullet$ min^{-1} = _____ METs

10. What is the caloric expenditure of a 155 lb. person exercising at 10 METs for 20 minutes on a Stairmaster? Assume 5 calories per liter of oxygen used.

    _____Kcals

Lab Nine
Resistance Training

Lab Nine corresponds to the following textbook readings:

Resistance Training Techniques	Chapter 19
Functional Training Concepts	Chapter 20

Lab Description

Resistance training is a vital component in the development of total fitness as muscular strength, endurance, and power are all related to function. The effects of participating in a regular resistance training program are far reaching, aiding in proper posture, the enhancements of joint and bone health, the facilitation of better movement economy, improved body composition, maintenance of proper function and independence, as well as decreasing the rate of muscle loss associated with aging (sarcopenia). This information suggests almost everyone can benefit from individually-appropriate resistance training activities.

As a competent personal trainer you must be able to understand the physiological effects of resistance training to the degree that you can explain the importance and benefits of this mode of exercise to clients. Additionally, key job tasks include: 1) competently designing and implementing a resistance training program based on client-specific goals, capabilities, and needs, 2) identifying, explaining, and demonstrating the correct biomechanical execution of resistance training exercises, 3) identifying appropriate starting points and instructing efficient skill acquisition and progressions, and 4) effectively utilizing the principles of specificity, overload, progression, and periodization. Competent personal trainers should be able to integrate resistance training for power, strength, and function for varying populations including children and the older adult.

Explored Procedures

- Perform biomechanical analysis of exercise movements
- Trunk musculature training exercises
- Upper body resistance training exercises
- Lower body resistance training exercises
- Functional training exercises and progressions

Lab Objectives

- Identify common movement errors and provide correction strategies
- Review and perform exercise activities for the trunk musculature
- Review and perform exercise activities for the upper body musculature
- Review and perform exercise activities for the lower body musculature
- Review and perform functional exercise activities
- Create functional training exercise progressions

Activity 9.1 Biomechanical Analysis

Activity Description

When moving the body under loaded conditions there is concern for soft tissue and joint health. Proper biomechanics are essential to injury-free training with resistance. The biomechanical factors of resistance training must be considered to prevent undesirable actions that are commonly performed with improper training technique due to poor or limited instruction. Most individuals, when left to their own accord, will perform resistance exercises incorrectly and through limited range of motion. Read the following overview before performing the lab activity to identify key areas of concern and common technique errors which should be addressed when instructing resistance training activities.

Pre-activity Review

Posture - Although weight training has a low occurrence of injury (about 4 per 1000 hours of participation), it does have the potential to cause or exacerbate specific biomechanical problems. The body is always under the influence of gravity ($9.81m/sec^2$) which dictates muscular contractions to counteract its constant pull. Whether performing actions in a standing or seated position, postural muscles must be activated to prevent the tendency to slouch or slump under gravitational pull. If gravity is not met by an equal and opposite muscular force, poor posture will result. Over time, compromised biomechanical positions can lead to overuse injuries and structural ROM changes. The same is true during acts of resistance training. The supportive joint structures and their associated musculature are at the greatest risk during loaded movements.

Under close analysis, the vertebral column is actually a combination support structure, protective nervous thoroughfare, and muscle attachment site. The overlapping structures are separated by sensitive discs and stabilized and controlled by the soft tissue that attaches to the spinous processes. The spine is constantly under the stress of maintaining posture, while working synergistically with muscle contractions to support movement. Due to the fact that this extended bony structure provides the framework for the central connecting component of the human body, it is important to maintain strength and joint integrity within the area.

Many muscles attach to the spine and indirectly affect its movement. For this reason, strength and ample ROM are necessary to allow the spine to correctly perform its role as a supportive structure. When the spine is not able to maintain its neutral position, there is usually associated stress caused by shearing or compressive forces. The resistive torques encountered during lifting can lead to back injury if not accounted for through proper joint biomechanics. Of particular concern are the joints formed between the two lowest lumbar vertebrae, L4 and L5 and L5 and S1 (the top of the sacrum). These joint formations have a high susceptibility to injury and are the site for most disc injuries. The primary reasons for this risk is the amount of torque created from the length of the resistance arm that is often applied during movements like the Back Squat, Romanian Deadlift, and the Good Morning exercise. In addition, this area experiences greater ROM requirements compared to other vertebral joints.

In lifting scenarios such as those mentioned above, the back muscles are forced to work with a low mechanical advantage. This requires greater force to accomplish the movement. In these situations, the intervertebral discs experience large amounts of compressive and rotational forces. Proper lifting posture and technique can alleviate some of the stress experienced, which in turn reduces the risk for injury. The back should never be loaded in the rounded position, nor axially loaded and rotated.

Neutral Spine or Flat Back - Neutral spine position entails maintaining the natural curvature of the spine (C1-C7 lordotic curve, T1-T12 kyphotic curve, L1-L5 lordotic curve, S1-S5 sacrum kyphotic curve) as seen in anatomical position. Neutral spine maximizes the efficiency of the natural structural alignment. Because the spine is involved in the execution of the majority of resistance training techniques, it is recommended that a person concentrate on keeping the spine in a neutral position to avoid disc shear, compression, and subsequent injury from incorrect back position. To accomplish this, clients should be taught proper lifting posture prior to performing movements under the stress of additional resistance. By assuming a neutral spine position and maintaining it through the movement, the lifter can create a safe internal lifting environment.

Shoulder Joint - The shoulder joint can be problematic under assignments of force application as well. Although a highly mobile joint structure, it is often vulnerable under stress in some of its functionally attainable positions. Unlike the ball and socket joint formed at the hip, the shoulder sits in a shallow cavity. This limited articulation allows for mobility at the sacrifice of stability. The main stability of the joint comes from three sets of ligaments and four muscles called the rotator cuff. Additional stability is added from the surrounding gross musculature and the particulars within the joint cavity. This stability network creates an extremely sensitive environment, which can be upset by any number of minor afflictions.

Any inflammation in the area increases the frictional coefficient of the related structures. This increased friction causes additional stress on the inflamed area, as well as the other soft tissues in the shoulder. Shoulders become increasingly problematic when they experience compromised stability due to an injury. Common contributing injury scenarios can be attributed to overuse, ballistic contractions, impingement, or high force application. Many fitness enthusiasts feel the pain signals indicating something is wrong, but opt to follow the old adage "no pain, no gain." Tendonitis, bursitis, impingement syndrome, dislocations, and the tearing of muscles, ligaments, and tendons can occur during weight training. Pressing exercises such as the flat bench, overhead press, and incline chest press cause severe stress on the joint and, if performed incorrectly or with an inappropriate load, can lead to debilitating injuries.

Note: Bench presses are of particular concern because normal scapular retractory movements can be inhibited by the bench. This movement limitation increases shoulder stress and is commonly linked to overuse injuries.

Since the glenohumeral joint is not a closed ball and socket, the shoulder is subject to elevated risk of injury when performing tasks while the humerus is externally rotated, abducted, and fully flexed. This condition causes the forces to be directed downward and sometimes backward upon an open joint capsule. In this position, the joint is at its greatest risk and resisted movements require significant strength and stability from soft tissue sources because the socket does not effectively support it. For this reason, extreme care should be taken when doing all pressing movements and correct biomechanics should always be adhered to. Additionally, pressing exercises should <u>never</u> be performed behind the head because of the increased risk that has them classified as contraindicated movements.

Preventive measures can be taken to ensure that joint health is maintained during the application of weight training programs. The first step is teaching proper training techniques and limiting exercises that place undue stress on the joint. All training movements should be properly controlled with particular attention to functional ROM and the avoidance of momentum forces, especially at directional transition. The shoulder should be trained using an exercise prescription that balances the musculature acting upon the joint to maintain its integrity. Rotator cuff strength and flexibility deserve specific attention in any program where resistance training is employed.

Knee Joint - The knee is another joint regularly stressed during movement and is susceptible to several types of injuries from resistance training. The most common mistake made during the performance of resistance training exercises aimed at leg development is in the position of the knee during sagittal movement. During activities such as the squat, leg press, lunge, and step-up, many lifters allow the knee to cross the plane of the toe. This causes tibial translation, which places additional stress on the joint and can lead to injury. Additionally, knee flexion beyond 90 degrees can produce similar detrimental forces.

Diagram below represents the dynamics of *tibial translation*

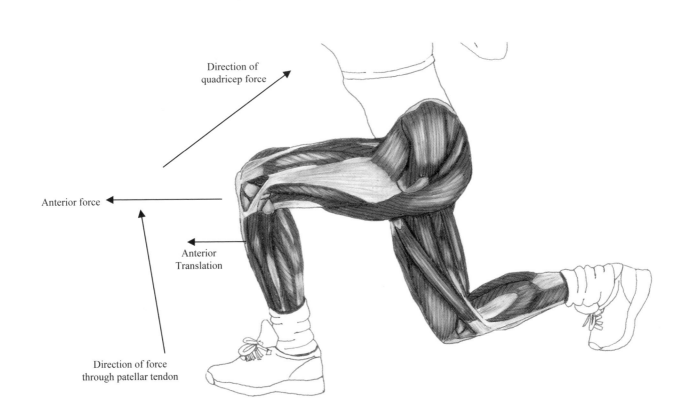

When the knee crosses the plane of the toes, the lifters center of gravity migrates forward. This produces ankle dorsi flexion and anterior tibial translation during the movement. Tibial translation is a concern because the tibia is pulled anteriorly putting stress on ligaments and joint structures.

Another area for concern arises when machines are used for lower body training. Many exercisers fail to align the joint axis of the machine with the joint axis of the body. This is commonly seen on the leg extension and flexion machines. Quite often the knee is shifted forward in front of the machine's axis of rotation, which increases the shear stress on the joint.

As the dynamics/intensity of the activity increases so does the risk for serious injuries. This is particularly true when the knee experiences forces from the frontal plane. Since the knee is a hinge joint designed to move in the sagittal plane, it is subject to injury during lateral and twisting movements. Activities that call for a rapid change of direction, as seen in plyometrics and agility drills, can increase the risk of ligament and cartilage injury.

Procedure

Analyze the following movements for biomechanical correctness. Identify the exercises that are performed correctly and those that are performed with biomechanical errors. Make recommendations to correct the exercises that are performed improperly. Chapter 2 can be referenced for assistance.

Lat Pulldown

Correct _____   Incorrect _____

Error: _____

_____

Correction: _____

_____

Front Raise

Correct _____   Incorrect _____

Error: _____

_____

Correction: _____

_____

Bent-Over Row

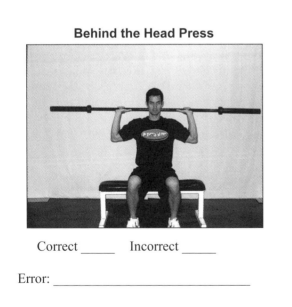

Correct _____   Incorrect _____

Error: _____

_____

Correction: _____

_____

Romanian Deadlift

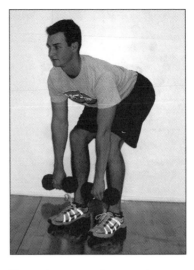

Correct _____   Incorrect _____

Error: _____

_____

Correction: _____

_____

Lunge

Behind the Head Press

Correct _____   Incorrect _____

Error: _____

_____

Correction: _____

_____

Correct _____   Incorrect _____

Error: _____

_____

Correction: _____

_____

Trunk Rotation

Leg Lifts

Correct _____   Incorrect _____

Error: _____

_____

Correction: _____

_____

Correct _____   Incorrect _____

Error: _____

_____

Correction: _____

_____

Activity 9.2 Trunk Musculature Resistance Training

Activity Description

The exercises presented within this section are intended to give the user a foundation for some basic resistance training movements for the trunk musculature. Although there are numerous exercises and exercise variations that can be utilized in a training program, the exercises performed in this activity cover the primary actions of the trunk including flexion, extension, lateral flexion, and rotation. Many of the movements can be performed using various resistance modalities (barbells, dumbbells, machines, tubing, cables, medicine balls, etc.), but for all intended purposes, there is little variation in the gross mechanical execution of each exercise regardless of the resistance used.

Procedures

Have a volunteer subject perform the following resistance training exercises under your guidance and supervision. Be sure to read the activity description in Chapter 19 of the course textbook and have a thorough understanding of each movement prior to the performance of the exercise. This is of extreme importance, as the personal trainer must have a comprehensive working knowledge of a multitude of training techniques which can be safely implemented into a resistance training program. Upon completion of this activity, participants should be able to properly describe, demonstrate, instruct, and spot each activity for new and experienced clients.

Example

Medicine Ball Abdominal Pullovers

Primary Joint Action: <u>Trunk flexion, shoulder extension</u>

Prime Mover: <u>Rectus abdominis, latissimus dorsi</u>

Assistive Movers: <u>Pectoralis major, iliopsoas, obliques</u>

Common Error: <u>Over acceleration of shoulder extension, anterior pelvic tilt during eccentric</u>

Exercise Variation: <u>Cable abdominal pullovers</u>

<u> X </u> Activity Performed

Abdominal Curl-up

Primary Joint Action: _____

Prime Mover: _____

Assistive Movers: _____

Common Error: _____

Exercise Variation: _____

_____ Activity Performed

Reverse Abdominal Curl-up

Primary Joint Action: _____

Prime Mover: _____

Assistive Movers: _____

Common Error: _____

Exercise Variation: _____

_____ Activity Performed

Physioball Curl-up

Primary Joint Action: _____

Prime Mover: _____

Assistive Movers: _____

Common Error: _____

Exercise Variation: _____

_____ Activity Performed

Alternating Ankle Touches

Primary Joint Action: _____

Prime Mover: _____

Assistive Movers: _____

Common Error: _____

Exercise Variation: _____

_____ Activity Performed

Floor Bridging

Primary Joint Action: _____

Prime Mover: _____

Assistive Movers: _____

Common Error: _____

Exercise Variation: _____

_____ Activity Performed

Opposite Raise

Primary Joint Action: _____

Prime Mover: _____

Assistive Movers: _____

Common Error: _____

Exercise Variation: _____

_____ Activity Performed

Physioball Back Extension

Primary Joint Action: _____

Prime Mover: _____

Assistive Movers: _____

Common Error: _____

Exercise Variation: _____

_____ Activity Performed

Medicine Ball Seated Reach

Primary Joint Action: _____

Prime Mover: _____

Assistive Movers: _____

Common Error: _____

Exercise Variation: _____

_____ Activity Performed

Good Morning

Primary Joint Action: _____

Prime Mover: _____

Assistive Movers: _____

Common Error: _____

Exercise Variation: _____

_____ Activity Performed

Seated Cable Chops

Primary Joint Action: _____

Prime Mover: _____

Assistive Movers: _____

Common Error: _____

Exercise Variation: _____

_____ Activity Performed

Physioball Roll-up

Primary Joint Action: _____

Prime Mover: _____

Assistive Movers: _____

Common Error: _____

Exercise Variation: _____

_____ Activity Performed

Activity 9.3 Upper Body Resistance Training

Activity Description

The exercises presented within this section are intended to give the user a foundation for some basic resistance training movements for the trunk musculature. Although there are numerous exercises and exercise variations that can be utilized, the exercises performed in this activity cover the primary actions of the upper body musculature. Consistent with the trunk activities, many of these movements can also be performed using various other resistance modalities (barbells, dumbbells, machines, tubing, cables, medicine balls, etc.), but again, there is little variation in the gross mechanical execution of each exercise.

Procedures

Have a volunteer subject perform the following resistance training exercises under your guidance and supervision. Be sure to read the activity description in Chapter 19 of the course textbook and have a thorough understanding of each movement prior to the performance of the exercise. At the completion of this activity, participants should be able to properly describe, demonstrate, instruct, and spot each activity for new and veteran clients.

Example
Bench Press

Primary Joint Action: Humeral horizontal adduction, elbow extension

Prime Mover: Pectoralis major

Assistive Movers: Anterior deltoid, triceps brachii

Common Error: Improper deceleration to chest, hip extension

Exercise Variation: Dumbbell bench press

Spotting Technique: Assisted lift-off, spot the bar, re-rack with alternate grip

_X_ Activity Performed

Incline Bench Press

Primary Joint Action: _____

Prime Mover: _____

Assistive Movers: _____

Common Error: _____

Exercise Variation: _____

Spotting Techniques: _____

_____ Activity Performed

Chest Flye

Primary Joint Action: _____

Prime Mover: _____

Assistive Movers: _____

Common Error: _____

Exercise Variation: _____

Spotting Techniques: _____

_____ Activity Performed

Bench Push-up

Primary Joint Action: _____

Prime Mover: _____

Assistive Movers: _____

Common Error: _____

Exercise Variation: _____

Spotting Techniques: _____

_____ Activity Performed

Dumbbell Shoulder Press

Primary Joint Action: _____

Prime Mover: _____

Assistive Movers: _____

Common Error: _____

Exercise Variation: _____

Spotting Techniques: _____

_____ Activity Performed

Upright Row

Primary Joint Action: _____

Prime Mover: _____

Assistive Movers: _____

Common Error: _____

Exercise Variation: _____

Spotting Techniques: _____

_____ Activity Performed

Lateral Deltoid Raise

Primary Joint Action: _____

Prime Mover: _____

Assistive Movers: _____

Common Error: _____

Exercise Variation: _____

Spotting Techniques: _____

_____ Activity Performed

Rear Deltoid Raise

Primary Joint Action: _____

Prime Mover: _____

Assistive Movers: _____

Common Error: _____

Exercise Variation: _____

Spotting Techniques: _____

_____ Activity Performed

Front Raise

Primary Joint Action: _____

Prime Mover: _____

Assistive Movers: _____

Common Error: _____

Exercise Variation: _____

Spotting Techniques: _____

_____ Activity Performed

Bent-Over Row

Primary Joint Action: _____

Prime Mover: _____

Assistive Movers: _____

Common Error: _____

Exercise Variation: _____

Spotting Techniques: _____

_____ Activity Performed

Seated Row

Primary Joint Action: _____

Prime Mover: _____

Assistive Movers: _____

Common Error: _____

Exercise Variation: _____

Spotting Techniques: _____

_____ Activity Performed

Lat Pull-down

Primary Joint Action: _____

Prime Mover: _____

Assistive Movers: _____

Common Error: _____

Exercise Variation: _____

Spotting Techniques: _____

_____ Activity Performed

Single Arm Row

Primary Joint Action: _____

Prime Mover: _____

Assistive Movers: _____

Common Error: _____

Exercise Variation: _____

Spotting Techniques: _____

_____ Activity Performed

Tricep Extension

Primary Joint Action: _____

Prime Mover: _____

Assistive Movers: _____

Common Error: _____

Exercise Variation: _____

Spotting Techniques: _____

_____ Activity Performed

Tricep Kickback

Primary Joint Action: _____

Prime Mover: _____

Assistive Movers: _____

Common Error: _____

Exercise Variation: _____

Spotting Techniques: _____

_____ Activity Performed

Tricep Bench Dips

Primary Joint Action: _____

Prime Mover: _____

Assistive Movers: _____

Common Error: _____

Exercise Variation: _____

Spotting Techniques: _____

_____ Activity Performed

Tricep Pushdown

Primary Joint Action: _____

Prime Mover: _____

Assistive Movers: _____

Common Error: _____

Exercise Variation: _____

Spotting Techniques: _____

_____ Activity Performed

Bicep Curl

Primary Joint Action: _____

Prime Mover: _____

Assistive Movers: _____

Common Error: _____

Exercise Variation: _____

Spotting Techniques: _____

_____ Activity Performed

Hammer Curls

Primary Joint Action: _____

Prime Mover: _____

Assistive Movers: _____

Common Error: _____

Exercise Variation: _____

Spotting Techniques: _____

_____ Activity Performed

Internal Rotator

Primary Joint Action: _____

Prime Mover: _____

Assistive Movers: _____

Common Error: _____

Exercise Variation: _____

Spotting Techniques: _____

_____ Activity Performed

External Rotator

Primary Joint Action: _____

Prime Mover: _____

Assistive Movers: _____

Common Error: _____

Exercise Variation: _____

Spotting Techniques: _____

_____ Activity Performed

The preceding exercises include some of the basic free weight movements that can be prescribed for your clients. They should not be viewed as the end-all to exercises for the upper body. They simply provide a small sampling of the activities that can be performed using free weights. The chart below illustrates some of the traditional variations of the previous exercises. They are segmented into different categories and provide you with a quick reference when putting together future resistance training programs.

Push-up Movements	90° Press Movements	Incline Press Movements
Push-up from the floor Push-up from knees Push-up on a bench Push-up with feet elevated Close grip push-up Push-up on a physioball from knees Push-up on a physioball legs straight Push-up on a physioball from one leg	Machine bench press Barbell bench press Close grip bench press Dumbbell (db) bench press Single arm db bench press Alternating single arm db bench press Barbell bench press on physioball DB bench press on physioball Standing chest press with tubing Alternating cable press	Machine incline press Barbell incline press Close grip incline press Dumbbell incline press Alternating single arm incline db bench press Incline barbell bench press on physioball Incline db bench press on physioball

Decline Press Movements	Flyes and Pullovers	Overhead Shoulder Presses
Machine decline press Barbell decline press Close grip decline press Dumbbell decline press Single arm db decline press Alternating single arm decline db bench press Standing cable decline press	Pec dec Machine flyes Machine pullover Flat bench dumbbell flyes Incline dumbbell flyes Decline dumbbell flyes Cable chest cross over Incline flyes on physioball Flat flyes on physioball	Machine shoulder press Seated barbell shoulder press Standing barbell shoulder press Seated dumbbell shoulder press Standing dumbbell shoulder press Seated mb overhead shoulder press Seated db shoulder press on physioball Seated alternating dumbbell shoulder press on physioball

Shoulder Raises	Upright Rows	Tricep Extensions
Dumbbell side lateral raise Single arm db side lateral raise Cable side lateral raise Theraband side lateral raise Single arm cable side lateral raise Dumbbell anterior raise Alternating db anterior raise Alternating db front/side raise Seated side lateral raise Seated on physioball side lateral raise DB bent over rear deltoid raise Supine lateral raise with band	Barbell upright row Dumbbell upright row Alternating dumbbell upright row Cable upright row Theraband upright row Wide grip upright row Single arm upright row Alternating db upright row Seated cable upright row	Standing tricep extension Supine tricep extension Single arm tricep extension Tricep pushdown Tricep dips Close grip press Tricep kickbacks Single arm cable extension

Pull-downs	Rows	Bicep Curls
Wide grip lat pull-downs Close grip lat pull-downs Parallel grip pull-downs Reverse grip pull-downs V-bar pull-down Seated on physioball pull-downs Single arm pull-downs Pull-ups Chin-ups	Wide grip cable rows Narrow grip cable rows Single arm cable row Single arm db row 2 arm cable row Bent over barbell rows Bent over db rows Bent over machine row Seated machine rows T-bar rows	Standing straight bar curl Standing db curl Seated db curl Alternating db curl Preacher curl Cable curl with bar One arm cable curl Reverse grip curl Hammer curl

Activity 9.4 Lower Body Resistance Training

Activity Description

Activity 9.4 presents lower body resistance training exercise techniques. When instructed correctly, almost all healthy participants can perform the exercises presented in this lab experience. A progressive continuum exists for each exercise, which enables the personal trainer to manipulate movements to fit the individual abilities of different clients. The goal of the resistance training lab is to focus on the proper instruction of exercise form and technique. If an individual cannot perform an exercise correctly, a modification can be made or a different exercise can be substituted in its place. Body alignment and mechanics are vital to safe and effective execution of movements under resistance. This makes recognizing and controlling proper body movements a pivotal skill for the personal trainer and should be a primary consideration in this lab experience.

Practicing the activities without weight or with very little resistance at the onset of the instruction will enable the subject to develop correct motor patterning and enhanced kinesthetic awareness. Skill acquisition and progressions should follow a building block approach to best acclimate the body for the next task. Using appropriate teaching cues and hands-on instruction will aid in the learning process. Joint alignment is particularly important with resistance training and should be closely monitored during each exercise.

Procedures

Have a volunteer subject perform the following resistance training exercises under your guidance and supervision. Be sure to read the activity description in Chapter 19 of the course textbook and have a thorough understanding of each movement prior to the performance of the exercise. This is of extreme importance as the personal trainer must have a comprehensive working knowledge of a multitude of training techniques and be able to properly describe, demonstrate, instruct, and spot each activity for new and veteran clients.

Example

Split Squat

Primary Joint Action: Hip extension, knee extension

Prime Mover: Gluteus Maximus, rectus femoris

Assistive Movers: Bicep femoris, vastus intermedius

Common Error: Knee crosses plane of toe, incomplete back leg flexion

Exercise Variation: Dumbbell split squat

X   Activity Performed

Back Squat

Primary Joint Action: _____

Prime Mover: _____

Assistive Movers: _____

Common Error: _____

Exercise Variation: _____

Spotting Techniques: _____

_____ Activity Performed

Modified Deadlift

Primary Joint Action: _____

Prime Mover: _____

Assistive Movers: _____

Common Error: _____

Exercise Variation: _____

Spotting Techniques: _____

_____ Activity Performed

Romanian Deadlift

Primary Joint Action: _____

Prime Mover: _____

Assistive Movers: _____

Common Error: _____

Exercise Variation: _____

Spotting Techniques: _____

_____ Activity Performed

Lunge

Primary Joint Action: _____

Prime Mover: _____

Assistive Movers: _____

Common Error: _____

Exercise Variation: _____

Spotting Techniques: _____

_____ Activity Performed

Lateral Lunge

Primary Joint Action: _____

Prime Mover: _____

Assistive Movers: _____

Common Error: _____

Exercise Variation: _____

Spotting Techniques: _____

_____ Activity Performed

Step-up

Primary Joint Action: _____

Prime Mover: _____

Assistive Movers: _____

Common Error: _____

Exercise Variation: _____

Spotting Techniques: _____

_____ Activity Performed

Single-leg Squat

Primary Joint Action: _____

Prime Mover: _____

Assistive Movers: _____

Common Error: _____

Exercise Variation: _____

Spotting Techniques: _____

_____ Activity Performed

Leg Press

Primary Joint Action: _____

Prime Mover: _____

Assistive Movers: _____

Common Error: _____

Exercise Variation: _____

Spotting Techniques: _____

_____ Activity Performed

Leg Curl

Primary Joint Action: _____

Prime Mover: _____

Assistive Movers: _____

Common Error: _____

Exercise Variation: _____

Spotting Techniques: _____

_____ Activity Performed

Leg Curl on Ball

Primary Joint Action: _____

Prime Mover: _____

Assistive Movers: _____

Common Error: _____

Exercise Variation: _____

Spotting Techniques: _____

_____ Activity Performed

Leg Extension

Primary Joint Action: _____

Prime Mover: _____

Assistive Movers: _____

Common Error: _____

Exercise Variation: _____

Spotting Techniques: _____

_____ Activity Performed

Calf Raise

Primary Joint Action: _____

Prime Mover: _____

Assistive Movers: _____

Common Error: _____

Exercise Variation: _____

Spotting Techniques: _____

_____ Activity Performed

The preceding exercises are some of the basic free weight movements that can be prescribed for your clients. They should not be viewed as the end-all to exercises for the lower body. They simply provide a small sampling of the activities that can be performed using free weights. The chart below illustrates many of the variations of the previous exercises. They are segmented into different categories and provide you with a quick reference when putting together future resistance training programs.

Lunge	Knee Extension	Knee Flexion
Stationary lunge (split squat) Forward lunge Forward walking lunge Side walking lunge 45 Degree stepping lunge Reverse or drop lunge Lunge on step Lunge with bar Lunge with medicine ball Overhead lunge Cable drop lunge Rear leg on ball lunge Lunge with foot on disk (stability) Dynamic Lunge (forward to backward) Lateral lunge	Leg extension machine Leg extension machine, single leg Seated physioball leg extension Manual resisted leg extension Step-ups Step-up with bar Step-up with a medicine ball Step-up with dumbbells Lateral step-ups High box step-up – body weight	Prone leg curl Manual leg curl Theraband leg curl Seated leg curl Single leg curl Leg curl on physioball Leg curl with cable Buddy hamstrings
Deadlift	**Hip Extension**	**Squat and Leg Press**
Regular deadlift with bar Dumbbell deadlift Modified deadlift with bar or db Sumo deadlift with bar or db Romanian deadlift (RDL) with bar Romanian deadlift with dumbbells Single leg RDL Cable deadlift	Reverse alternating leg raise Hip extension (bridge) Single leg hip extension Machine hip extension Cable hip extension	Squat Bar squat Dumbbell squat Medicine ball squat Front squat Sumo squat (wide stance) Single leg squat with bar Single leg squat with dumbbell Leg press Single leg press
Plantar Flexion	**Dorsi Flexion**	**Hip Adduction/Abduction**
Standing calf raise Seated calf raise Machine plantar flexion	Toe raises Seated dorsi flexion with bands Machine dorsi flex	Side lunge Wide squat 4-way hip machine Cable adduction Cable abduction

Activity 9.5 Functional Resistance Training

Activity Description

Most traditional exercises have limited carry-over to improvements in real world applications due to the stable linear production of force in a single plane. Although ideal for hypertrophy training, which aims to isolate target tissue and maximize the recruitment of fibers, traditional resistance training exercises do very little for neuromuscular efficiency in other tasks. Traditional resistance training does increase strength within the specific movement, but again, very few actions performed in sports and everyday life are stable, bilateral, and single plane-linear. Most resistance training exercises allow for direct acceleration with limited offsetting forces which cause improvements in strength specific to the action, but how often does one duplicate the bench pressing action in a day? Rarely are people lying on the ground with a need to lift a heavy object directly above their chest. Most activities are ground based, closed-chain, and asymmetrically loaded. Carrying a child or clothing basket up a flight of stairs is not duplicated on a leg extension machine, nor does seated row emulate the stabilization and pulling action of opening a heavy door. Most personal training client's will not be bodybuilders or compete at lifting competitions and therefore program focus should reflect this fact. Personal training program activities should encourage improvements in ground reaction forces transferred through the tibia to varying kinetic chains. Challenging the central nervous system using unloaded and loaded motor patterns creates improvements in neural coordination. The neuromuscular enhancements cause harmonious and synchronized actions which lead to improved efficiency in everyday tasks.

Procedures: Part One

Modifying traditional lifts to exercises aimed at improving function simply requires increasing the neuromuscular demands. This can be done by performing the activities in a standing position, changing the stability requirements via center of gravity adjustments, asymmetrically loading and/or modifying the contact surface stability, as well as using complex movements and multiple planes. Review the following exercises in Chapter 20 and complete the activities listed below. After completing the functional training activities, complete the tables that follow.

Lateral asymmetrically loaded step-up

__X__ Activity Performed

Planes of motion involved: <u>Sagittal-frontal</u>

Movement actions: <u>Knee extension, hip extension, hip adduction</u>

How is stability challenged? <u>Asymmetrical load, center of gravity raised and line of gravity moved towards the terminal end of the base of support, stability lost and regained over a smaller base of support</u>

Lunge with trunk rotation

_____ Activity Performed

Planes of motion involved: _____

Movement actions: _____

How is stability challenged? _____

Reverse lunge with asymmetrical band or cable row

_____ Activity Performed

Planes of motion involved: _____

Movement actions: _____

How is stability challenged? _____

Forward-diagonal lunge with single arm band punch

_____ Activity Performed

Planes of motion involved: _____

Movement actions: _____

How is stability challenged? _____

Single leg-single arm dumbbell Romanian deadlift

_____ Activity Performed

Planes of motion involved: _____

Movement actions: _____

How is stability challenged? _____

Push-ups on a physioball

_____ Activity Performed

Planes of motion involved: _____

Movement actions: _____

How is stability challenged? _____

Single arm overhead squat

_____ Activity Performed

Planes of motion involved: _____

Movement actions: _____

How is stability challenged? _____

Procedures: Part Two

Understanding how to integrate the functional exercise into a traditional program can be done relatively easily as long as there is a basic understanding of the movement and the muscle groups involved. In the following activity you will be asked to transfer your knowledge of traditional training modalities into more functional exercises by converting the listed exercises into activities that address the same muscle group, but with additional stability and integration.

Examples

Standing cable torso twist	Cable torso twist in isometric lunge stance
Push-up on floor	Push-up with hands or feet on physioball
Forward lunge	Forward lunge with diagonal medicine ball chop
Bench press	Single arm alternating press on physioball
Back squat	Medicine ball overhead squat on stability discs
High row	Modified pull-up with feet on physioball
Low row	Single leg stance band row
Leg curls	Supine leg curls with feet on physioball
Side lateral raise	Asymmetrical raise seated on ball with one foot elevated

Traditional	Functional
Bench press	Example: Seated band chest press on ball or Push-ups on the ball
Back squat	
Seated cable row	
Romanian deadlift	
Shoulder side raise	
Leg curls	
Ab crunch	
Lunges	
Torso twists	

Procedures: Part Three

Once a traditional exercise has been mastered, it can be progressed into more challenging activities. Functional progressions utilize many more variables than traditional weight lifting where the most common progression is with adjustments to resistance. Considering neuromuscular adaptation rates and realistic performance capability adjustments, progress the following exercises in a functional manner. There may be numerous correct responses, but any adjustment decision must be logical and appropriate for the client.

Example

Exercise.	Static Lunge – Skill acquisition
Progression 1.	Walking lunge – Dynamic
Progression 2.	Walking lunge with dumbbells – Resisted dynamic
Progression 3.	Medicine ball overhead walking lunge – Raised center of gravity
Progression 4.	Lunge with medicine ball trunk rotation – Multiplaner

Exercise   Seated Band Chest Press – Skill acquisition

Progression 1. _____

Progression 2. _____

Progression 3. _____

Progression 4. _____

Exercise   Push-up – Skill acquisition

Progression 1. _____

Progression 2. _____

Progression 3. _____

Progression 4. _____

Exercise   Standing Band Row – Skill acquisition

Progression 1. _____

Progression 2. _____

Progression 3. _____

Progression 4. _____

Lab Nine Submission Form – Resistance Training

1. What is the correct course of action if your client is having difficulty controlling the weights throughout the ROM in the Dumbbell Bench Press exercise?

_____

_____

2. Why should behind the head pressing and pulling activities be avoided?

_____

_____

3. _____ pelvic tilt should precede abdominal flexion exercises.

4. Identify the type of contraction taking place in the muscles below during the descent of the back squat exercise.

A. Vastus Lateralis: _____

B. Erector Spinae: _____

C. Gluteus Maximus: _____

5. Your new client is having difficulty keeping the knees from tracking over the toes during the execution of a lunge. What can a trainer say or do to help the client with proper technique adherence?

_____

_____

_____

6. What adjustments can be made if a client is experiencing excessive travel of the knee over the toes (breaking the plane of the toes) during the leg press exercise?

_____

_____

Lab Nine Submission Form – Resistance Training

7. When is trunk rotation contraindicated due to biomechanical stress?

_____

_____

8. Provide three (3) functional progressions for the Romanian deadlift.

       1. _____

       2. _____

       3. _____

9. Why is the supine leg lift contraindicated?

_____

_____

10. When is the shoulder at the greatest risk for injury?

_____

Lab Ten
Resistance Training Programming

Lab Ten corresponds to the following textbook reading:

Creating an Exercise Program   Chapter 21

Lab Description
Exercise programming is the cornerstone of the personal trainer's job responsibilities. The design of a comprehensive program requires a thorough understanding of the specific energy systems' work capabilities, relationship of stress and duration to fatigue, and recovery or replenishment requirements necessary to accommodate demands. It must correctly apply the principles of exercise in a manner that produces the right stress, in appropriate dosage, for the necessary period of time, with adequate frequency to create progressive and desired adaptational responses. It is further complicated as personal training services are usually offered 2-3 days per week and must elicit a training response from numerous health and fitness components simultaneously, while working within the capabilities of the client. Although programming is a seemingly difficult task, there are numerous anaerobic and aerobic training systems that can be leveraged to help maximize the efficiency of the training. Integrating these concepts into a program matrix will increase the likelihood of success from personal training services.

Explored Procedures
- Application of the principles of exercise programming
- Components of program design
- Implementation of resistance training systems and programming options
- Exercise selection for client specific needs
- Circuit training exercise prescription

Lab Objectives
- Understand how the principles of exercise are linked to physiological adaptations
- Understand the variables that make up correct program design
- Identify appropriate starting points for intensity and duration based on quantified individual physiological parameters
- Understand the relationship between intensity, rest interval, and adaptation outcomes
- Successfully prescribe exercise based on individual findings

---

Activity 10.1 Principles and Systems of Resistance Training Programming

Activity Description – Programming Part One
In order to properly prescribe exercises and create effective programs, the principles of exercise must be appropriately applied within the training activities. The correct *application* of these principles and terms is necessary to cause adaptations, maximize program effectiveness, and to avoid injury. This section will identify the key program components and how they are applied within an exercise prescription.

Exercise Order
Although there are countless training exercises and varying performance techniques, there are some simple rules that can be applied to help formulate the exercise prescription as it relates to exercise order. It is important to understand that these guidelines are general in scope and should not be viewed as the end all to resistance training programming as individual factors may warrant additional consideration or adjustments.

Recommended Exercise Order

- Complex movements (multi-joint) to simple movements (single joint)

- High skill level to low skill level or unstable to stable

- Multiplane movements to single plane movements

- Large muscle groups to small muscle groups

- Fast movements to slow movements

- High intensity to low intensity

Note: If deficiencies exist, they should be addressed as a priority in the exercise prescription and may precede the above order recommendations. Additionally, the programming should reflect the needs analysis, which is based on exercise assessment results and goals.

Procedures

Proper exercise order is a relevant part of the total exercise prescription. The following groups of exercises are not in proper order. Place them in the appropriate order, keeping in mind the standard principles of order. Assume each exercise is performed to volitional failure using 8-10 repetitions (~75%-80% 1RM).

A

1. Leg Extension   _____

2. Calf Raise   _____

3. Squat   _____

4. Step-up   _____

B

1. Flyes   _____

2. Bicep Curls   _____

3. Bench Press   _____

4. Tricep Extension   _____

C

1. Romanian Deadlift   _____

2. Leg Press   _____

3. Leg Extension   _____

4. Barbell Side Lunges _____

5. Weighted Squat Jump _____

D

1. Dumbbell Incline Press _____

2. Tricep Kickback   _____

3. Side Lateral Raises   _____

4. Single Arm Rows   _____

5. Deadlift   _____

Rest Intervals

Procedures

Rest intervals are necessary for the rephosphorylation of ATP, the management of hydrogen ions, as well as determining the resultant hormonal response to the stress of exercise. Specific rest intervals optimize the adaptation process and must be considered for the proper implementation of exercise programs. Incorrect rest intervals change the perception of stress and modify the outcome. Personal trainers must identify the rest interval required for the desired outcome and understand the relationship between the energy system and the work to rest ratio. Complete the following table by entering the correct information for the specific goal or outcome.

Intended Outcome	Activity	Energy System	Rest interval
Example: Aerobic conditioning	Cardio-circuit	Aerobic/glycolytic	Transitional rest <15 sec
Hypertrophy	Bicep curls 10 reps		
Strength	Back squats 6 reps		
Anaerobic endurance	Push-ups 25 reps		
Anaerobic power	Box jumps 6 reps		

Procedures

The key principles of exercise include specificity, overload, and progression. In many cases, the latter are combined to form progressive overload. Each holds particular merit in the design of an exercise program. Review the following definitions and complete the activity questions that follow.

Principle of Specificity

As the name implies, specificity refers to the goal-oriented outcome of a particular action or activity. In the case of resistance-training, the training effect is specific to the physiological systems used and method of overload employed during the training. Programs should have goal-oriented outcomes and the exercises employed must be specific to the attainment of the desired goals. For example, a person looking to increase power output would not gain performance benefits by performing high repetition training in a slow controlled manner. Likewise, muscle size and strength are specific to the muscle groups and muscle fibers recruited and overloaded. The exercises, intensity, and volume must be specific to the desired outcome.

Training specificity is the key to the proper effect of the exercise. Review the following training goals and place the letter that corresponds to the appropriate exercise selection identified as *specific* to the intended goal. Some of the activities will not be used to attend to the goals, therefore pick the best selection of the activities listed.

Goal	Activity
_____ Reduced tricep fat	a. Tricep extensions
_____ Increased closed-chain trunk stabilization	b. Romanian deadlift
_____ Hamstring strengthening	c. Chair stands
_____ Gluteus maximus ROM	d. Single leg squat
_____ Frontal plane, closed-chain movement proficiency	e. Squat to single arm dumbbell press
_____ Test for power in an older adult	f. High box step-up
_____ Dynamic flexibility for the hip flexor	g. 20 minutes interval training
	h. Lateral lunge
	i. Bench press
	j. 15 minutes steady-state 60% VO$_2$max

Principle of Overload

Overload is defined as a stress level beyond that to which the body is presently accustomed. It is the sole reason that the body adapts to exercise. Adaptations will occur as long as the physiological systems experience new perceived stress. Once the stress no longer exceeds the current level that the body is accustomed to, the adaptations will subside. This explains why people may workout for a period of time, and not make any new gains from the previous training period. If the body does not experience any new stress greater than that by which it is normally accustomed, no new adaptations will occur.

Procedures

Identifying the proper quantity of overload is necessary for progressive adaptation response. Insufficient stress or excessive stress will not create the desired outcome from the training. Personal trainers must recognize the different options that create overload for their clients while staying within the appropriate confines of ability and exercise tolerance. Select the appropriate overload for the exercises below.

Goal: Increase upper body strength

Exercise: Physioball dumbbell chest press

Overload options:

a. Increase resistance from 25 lbs. to 30 lbs.

b. Decrease rest interval from 60 seconds to 30 seconds

c. Perform exercise with single leg balance

d. Increase repetitions from 10 to 12

Goal: Increase shoulder hypertrophy

Exercise: Shoulder press

Overload options:

a. Increase resistance from 20 lbs. to 25 lbs. and decrease repetitions to 6

b. Perform pressing one arm at a time

c. Superset the exercise with side raise

d. Decrease weight to 15 lbs. increase the repetitions from 10 to 14

Goal: Increased total body function

Exercise: Lunge with a 10 lb. medicine ball

Overload options:

a. Switch to heavier resistance

b. Decrease weight and add trunk rotation

c. Increase repetitions to 20

d. Reduce rest interval from 45 seconds to 15 seconds

Goal: Increase leg power

Exercise: Squat

Overload options:

a. Increase weight from 135 lbs to 145 lbs.

b. Decrease rest interval from 90 seconds to 60 seconds

c. Increase the repetitions from 8 to 10

d. Switch to dumbbell squat jumps

Principle of Progression

The principle of progression by definition, is quite basic, but many programs fail because it is not effectively incorporated into the exercise design. Progression is simply the planned application of the overload principle. Applying progressive overload throughout a training cycle allows the body to adapt to the stress and improve. The improvement may be neural, biochemical, structural, or all three. For continual improvement over a time segment, the overload must be thoughtfully considered. A general recommendation is to increase the overload by 2.5%-5% once a repeated performance in two consecutive training sessions of the previous goal weight or stress is attained.

Procedures

Regardless of the type of training program you wish to prescribe, you must choose the appropriate starting points and exercise program progression for the client. The selection of the appropriate starting points and progressions will be based primarily on assessments, observations, and client feedback. Having a thorough understanding of the specific demands of a multitude of training techniques will enable you to adjust a client's routine to better accommodate individual abilities and the rate of physiological adaptations. Identify and select the appropriate movement progression from the starting points listed below.

Exercise starting point: <u>Box step-ups</u>

a. Holding dumbbells at side

b. Holding medicine ball overhead

c. Step-up with plyometric jump

d. Holding bar across shoulders

Exercise starting point: <u>Seated row</u>

a. Switch to bent-over row

b. Perform one arm at a time

c. Switch to modified pull-up

d. Increase range of motion

Exercise starting point: <u>Body weight squat</u>

a. Hold a medicine ball at chest height

b. Hold a bar across the shoulders

c. Widen the stance

d. Perform squat jumps

Exercise starting point: <u>Static lunge</u>

a. Switch to dynamic single step lunge

b. Switch to walking lunge

c. Perform reverse lunge

d. Hold dumbbells overhead

Exercise starting point: <u>Good morning exercise</u>

a. Place bar across shoulders

b. Perform on single leg

c. Hold medicine ball overhead

d. Hold 5 lb. weight against chest

Activity Description – Programming Part Two

Exercise prescription for personal training clients rely on creative, but logical strategies to apply adequate training stress in limited periods of time. The application of training systems allow for different types of program dynamics aimed at a variety of adaptational responses in a single exercise regimen. Utilizing the systems properly and in conjunction with the exercise and program principles allows for more efficient goal attainment than traditional set-rep schemes. The next section reviews the different training systems so they are properly understood for effective exercise programming.

Procedures

Training principles can be further employed using anaerobic and aerobic training systems. The systems allow for the application of progressive overload specific to the desired outcome. Complete the table by identifying the type of system utilized and the specific outcome that it is designed to meet.

Systems of Training

- Supersets
- Tri-sets
- Pyramid sets
- Circuits
- Complex
- Contrast

Training System	Activity	Rest Interval	Goal of Training
Example: Superset	10 repetitions of lat pull-down immediately followed by cable pullovers for 10 repetitions	30-60 seconds	Hypertrophy
	5 repetitions of squats immediately followed by 12 squat jumps	2 minutes following system	
	Seven exercises performed sequentially	Transitional period	
	Deadlift 7 reps, immediately followed by chest press of 8 reps, immediately followed by modified pull-up to failure	2 minutes following system	
	Leg press 10 reps using 75% 1RM - rest interval 8 reps using 80% 1RM - rest interval 6 reps using 85% 1RM	90 seconds	

Exercise Selection
Procedures

Proper exercise selection, particularly during the initial program design, is an important part of the total exercise prescription. The following activity requires you to review the sample case study and decide whether or not the listed exercise may be an appropriate selection for the initial training prescription. After making a decision to include the exercise or not, defend the rationale for your answer in the space provided. You may modify the exercise in your justification to include it in the program.

Sample Subject

Bob is a 49 year-old sedentary male. He is six feet tall and weighs 200 lbs. with a body composition of 20%. He complains of intermittent low back pain and has hypertension, but has been cleared for exercise. His fitness evaluation scores are as follows:

Push-up:	5
Ab-curl:	10 - difficulty maintaining posterior pelvic tilt
Squat:	Cannot perform technique properly
VO$_2$max:	29 ml $\cdot$ kg^{-1} $\cdot$ min^{-1}
Flexibility:	Tight hamstrings, tight glutes, tight upper back, poor shoulder flexion
Movement efficiency:	Has poor movement skills
Goal:	Overall improvement in health and fitness

Exercise	Yes/No	Why? – Defend your Answer
Back squat with bar		
Walking lunges with dumbbells		
Leg press		
RDL with bar		
Leg extension		
Lateral lunge		
Supine tricep extension		
Seated shoulder press with bar		
Seated row		
Close grip bench		
Deadlift		
Back extensions		
Push-ups from floor		

Exercise Prescription

Procedures

Exercise prescriptions require many considerations to be properly formulated. Depending on the individual's goals and fitness needs, the prescription should reflect their current fitness status, abilities, and availability of time. Personal training for results can be difficult with all the needs most clients have and the limited amount of time available to fit it all in. The following activity requires you to create a prescription overview that identifies when each muscle group will be trained (frequency).

Sample Subject

Suzie is a 33 year-old female. She is 5'7" tall and weighs 140 lbs. She is interested in improving her fitness level and toning her muscles. She is able to workout three days a week for an hour on Monday, Tuesday, and Thursday, but is willing to perform aerobic activity without your supervision. Using her data, create a general model for her exercise program by placing the muscle groups in the table to create her basic exercise model.

Body composition:	28%
Modified push-up:	9
Modified pull-up:	7
Abdominal curl-up:	20
Anaerobic step 1 min:	307 watts (50th percentile)

The minimum training parameter is for each muscle group is to be trained at least twice per week. Make appropriate considerations for recovery (rest).

Chest	Biceps
Shoulders	Quadriceps
Triceps	Hamstrings
Low Back	Aerobic Activity
Back (lats, rhomboids, trapezius)	Calves
Abdominals	Adductors

Sunday	Monday	Tuesday

Wednesday	Thursday	Friday	Saturday

Circuit Training

Procedures

Circuit training is an excellent method for eliciting several health responses using resistance training in a relatively short period of time. It can provide a great avenue for caloric expenditure, cardiovascular and strength benefits, as well as increasing volume with limited time availability. Create a circuit training program for the following individual.

Age:	42
Gender:	Male
Body Composition:	23%
Activity Level:	Previously sedentary
Goal:	Improved health
Time Constraints:	Subject has 30 minutes 3 days/week

Intensity: _____% (1RM)

Frequency: _____ days/week

Work Interval: _____ (Sec)

Rest Interval: _____ (Sec)

No. of Stations: _____

Time for Completion: _____ (1 Circuit)

No. of Circuits/Session: _____

Exercise selection in the order of the circuit

1. _____

2. _____

3. _____

4. _____

5. _____

6. _____

7. _____

8. _____

9. _____

10. _____

11. _____

12. _____

Procedures

For the same individual, provide a single-day excerpt of a three-day strength training program. The subject has engaged in your circuit program for four weeks and has been re-assessed for strength. His re-test values indicate he is ready to advance to more challenging activities. Based on his new goal of added strength, proper progression dictates allowing him to participate in a more comprehensive strength program. Fill in the boxes on the following chart to create his single-day workout. Assume a warm-up and cooldown are already included.

Exercise	Sets/Reps	Intensity	Rest Period
1.			
2.			
3.			
4.			
5.			
6.			
7.			
8.			

Lab Ten Submission Form – Resistance Training Programming

1. Define the following principles of exercise and provide an example of each.

Specificity: _____

_____

Example: _____

Overload: _____

_____

Example: _____

Progression: _____

_____

Example: _____

2. What is the appropriate progressive overload for increasing resistance of an exercise? _____ % per week

3. Place the exercises in the appropriate order by numbering the activities from 1-6. Assume all exercises are performed using 70% 1RM intensity.

_____ Romanian deadlift

_____ Pull-ups

_____ Back squat

_____ Bicep curl

_____ Seated row

_____ Calf raise

4. Identify the appropriate rest interval for the following training goals.

Hypertrophy: _____

Strength: _____

Endurance: _____

5. Identify the appropriate resistance training system based on the goal-intended outcome listed below.

    <u>**Goal Outcome**</u>

    Weight loss: _____

    Increasing vertical jump: _____

    Increasing maximal bench press: _____

6. For basic strength training, how many times per week should a muscle group be trained? _____

7. Provide a superset for the following goals, including the exercises and repetitions.

Hypertrophy

    Exercise 1. _____ Repetitions _____

    Exercise 2. _____ Repetitions _____

Strength

    Exercise 1. _____ Repetitions _____

    Exercise 2. _____ Repetitions _____

Endurance

    Exercise 1. _____ Repetitions _____

    Exercise 2. _____ Repetitions _____

8. Provide an example of an upper body contrast training exercise combination.

    Exercise 1. _____ Repetitions _____

    Exercise 2. _____ Repetitions _____

9. Provide an example of the pyramid training system for improving strength in the squat movement assuming the 1RM for the squat is 200 lbs.

	Resistance used	Repetitions
Set 1.	_____	_____
Set 2.	_____	_____
Set 3.	_____	_____
Set 4.	_____	_____

10. Write an eight (8) exercise circuit using only dumbbells and a physioball as the available equipment.

1. _____

2. _____

3. _____

4. _____

5. _____

6. _____

7. _____

8. _____

METS	CATEGORY	SPECIFIC ACTIVITY	METS	CATEGORY	SPECIFIC ACTIVITY
8.5	Bicycling	Bicycling, BMX, or mountain	5.5	Home Activities	Scrubbing floors
4.0	Bicycling	Bicycling, 10 mph, general	4.0	Home Activities	Sweeping garage, sidewalk
6.0	Bicycling	Bicycling, 10-11.9 mph	7.0	Home Activities	Carrying boxes
8.0	Bicycling	Bicycling, 12-13.9 mph	3.5	Home Activities	Standing-packing/unpacking
10.0	Bicycling	Bicycling, 14-15.9 mph	3.0	Home Activities	Putting away household items
12.0	Bicycling	Bicycling 16-19 mph	9.0	Home Activities	Move items upstairs
16.0	Bicycling	Bicycling .20 mph	2.5	Home Activities	Pumping gas
5.0	Conditioning	Stationary bicycle, general	3.0	Home Activities	Walking, noncleaning
3.0	Conditioning	Stationary bicycle, 50 W	2.5	Home Activities	Sitting-playing with child
5.5	Conditioning	Stationary bicycle, 100 W	2.8	Home Activities	Playing with child, light
7.0	Conditioning	Stationary bicycle, 150 W	4.0	Home Activities	Playing with child, moderate
10.5	Conditioning	Stationary bicycle, 200 W	5.0	Home Activities	Playing with child, vigorous
12.5	Conditioning	Stationary bicycle, 250 W	3.0	Home Activities	Child care
8.0	Conditioning	Calisthenics, heavy, vigorous	4.5	Home Repair	Automobile body work
4.5	Conditioning	Calisthenics, light, moderate	3.0	Home Repair	Automobile repair
8.0	Conditioning	Circuit Training, general	3.0	Home Repair	Carpentry, general, workshop
6.0	Conditioning	Weight lifting, vigorous effort	6.0	Home Repair	Carpentry, outside house
5.5	Conditioning	Health club exercise, general	5.0	Home Repair	Cleaning gutters
6.0	Conditioning	Stair-treadmill ergometer	5.0	Home Repair	Hanging storm windows
9.5	Conditioning	Rowing/ergometer/general	4.5	Home Repair	Laying/removing carpet
3.5	Conditioning	Rowing, 50 W, light effort	4.5	Home Repair	Laying tile
7.0	Conditioning	Rowing, 100 W, moderate	5.0	Home Repair	Painting
8.5	Conditioning	Rowing, 150 W, vigorous	6.0	Home Repair	Roofing
12.0	Conditioning	Rowing, 200 W, very vigorous	4.5	Home Repair	Scrape/paint boat
9.5	Conditioning	Ski machine, general	4.5	Home Repair	Wash, wax boat, car
4.0	Conditioning	Stretching, hatha yoga	3.0	Home Repair	Wiring, plumbing
6.0	Conditioning	Teaching aerobic class	0.9	Inactivity, Quiet	Lying quietly
4.0	Conditioning	Water aerobics/calisthenics	1.0	Inactivity, Quiet	Sitting quietly
3.0	Conditioning	Weight lifting light/general	0.9	Inactivity, Quiet	Sleeping
1.0	Conditioning	Whirl pool, sitting	1.2	Inactivity, Quiet	Standing quietly
6.0	Dancing	Aerobic, ballet/modern twist	1.0	Inactivity, Light	Recline-writing
6.0	Dancing	Aerobic general	1.0	Inactivity, Light	Recline-talking
5.0	Dancing	Aerobic low impact	1.0	Inactivity, Light	Recline-reading
7.0	Dancing	Aerobic high impact	5.5	Lawn & Garden	Mowing lawn, general
4.5	Dancing	General	2.5	Lawn & Garden	Riding mower
5.5	Dancing	Ballroom, fast	6.0	Lawn & Garden	Mowing lawn; hand mower
3.0	Dancing	Ballroom, slow	4.0	Lawn & Garden	Raking lawn
4.0	Fishing/Hunting	Fishing general	2.5	Lawn & Garden	Walking, applying fertilizer
2.5	Fishing/Hunting	Fishing from boat, sitting	1.5	Lawn & Garden	Watering garden
5.0	Fishing/Hunting	Hunting, general	5.0	Lawn & Garden	Gardening, general
2.5	Home Activities	Sweeping carpet/floors	3.0	Lawn & Garden	Picking up yard, light
4.5	Home Activities	Cleaning, heavy, vigorous	1.5	Miscellaneous	Playing cards, board games
3.5	Home Activities	Cleaning, general	1.8	Miscellaneous	Sitting-studying, general
2.5	Home Activities	Cleaning, light, moderate	1.8	Miscellaneous	Sitting-in class, general
2.3	Home Activities	Washing dishes	1.8	Miscellaneous	Standing-reading
2.5	Home Activities	Cooking	1.8	Music Playing	Accordion
2.5	Home Activities	Putting away groceries	2.0	Music Playing	Cello, flute, horn, woodwind
8.0	Home Activities	Carrying groceries upstairs	2.0	Music Playing	Guitar, classical, folk
3.5	Home Activities	Grocery shopping with cart	3.0	Music Playing	Guitar, rock band (standing)
2.0	Home Activities	Standing-shopping	2.5	Music Playing	Conducting, piano
2.3	Home Activities	Walking-shopping	2.5	Music Playing	Trumpet, violin
2.3	Home Activities	Ironing	4.0	Music Playing	Drums
1.5	Home Activities	Sitting, knitting, sewing	3.5	Music Playing	Trombone
2.0	Home Activities	Standing laundry	4.0	Music Playing	Marching band, baton twirling
2.0	Home Activities	Making bed	4.0	Occupation	Bakery, general
6.0	Home Activities	Moving furniture	2.3	Occupation	Bookbinding

METS	CATEGORY	SPECIFIC ACTIVITY	METS	CATEGORY	SPECIFIC ACTIVITY
6.0	Occupation	Building road	2.0	Self-Care	Bathing (sitting)
2.0	Occupation	Directing traffic	2.5	Self-Care	Dressing, undressing
3.5	Occupation	Carpentry, general	1.5	Self-Care	Eating (sitting)
8.0	Occupation	Carrying heavy loads	2.0	Self-Care	Talking & eating (standing)
8.0	Occupation	Carrying loads upstairs	2.5	Self-Care	Sitting or standing-grooming
5.5	Occupation	Construction, remodeling	4.0	Self-Care	Showering, toweling off
3.5	Occupation	Electrical work, plumbing	1.5	Sexual Activity	Active, vigorous effort
5.5	Occupation	Farming, shoveling grain	1.3	Sexual Activity	General, moderate effort
12.0	Occupation	Firefighter, general	1.0	Sexual Activity	Passive, light effort
8.0	Occupation	Forestry, general	4.5	Sports	Badminton, general
6.0	Occupation	Horse grooming	6.0	Sports	Basketball, general
3.5	Occupation	Locksmith	2.5	Sports	Billiards
3.0	Occupation	Machine tooling, welding	3.0	Sports	Bowling
7.0	Occupation	Masonry, concrete	12.0	Boxing	Boxing, in ring, general
1.5	Occupation	Sitting-light office work	5.0	Sports	Children's games, hopscotch
2.5	Occupation	Sitting, moderate	4.0	Sports	Coaching
2.5	Occupation	Standing, light/moderate	5.0	Sports	Cricket (batting, bowling)
3.5	Occupation	Standing, moderate	2.5	Sports	Croquet
4.0	Occupation	Standing moderate, heavy	4.0	Sports	Curling
8.0	Occupation	Steel mill, working in general	2.5	Sports	Darts
2.5	Occupation	Tailoring, general	6.0	Sports	Drag racing
6.5	Occupation	Truck driving, load/unload	6.0	Sports	Fencing
1.5	Occupation	Typing	8.0	Sports	Football, touch, flag, general
6.0	Occupation	Using heavy power tools	3.0	Sports	Frisbee, general
2.0	Occupation	Walking on job, <2.0mph	4.5	Sports	Golf, general
3.5	Occupation	Walking on job, 3.0mph	4.0	Sports	Gymnastics, general
4.0	Occupation	Walking on job, 3.5mph	4.0	Sports	Hacky sack
3.0	Occupation	Walking, 2.5mph, <25lb load	12.0	Sports	Handball, general
4.0	Occupation	Walking, 3.0mph, <25lb load	3.5	Sports	Hang gliding
4.5	Occupation	Walking, 3.5mph, <25lb load	8.0	Sports	Hockey, general
5.0	Occupation	Walking, 25-49lb load	4.0	Sports	Horseback riding, general
6.5	Occupation	Walking, 50-74lb load	10.0	Sports	Martial arts, general
7.5	Occupation	Walking, 75-99lb load	4.0	Sports	Juggling
8.5	Occupation	Walking, >=100lb load	7.0	Sports	Kickball
3.0	Occupation	Working in scene shop	8.0	Sports	Lacrosse
6.0	Running	Jog/walk combination	4.0	Sports	Moto-cross
7.0	Running	Jogging, general	6.0	Sports	Paddleball, general
8.0	Running	Running, 5mph	8.0	Sports	Polo
9.0	Running	Running, 5.2mph	7.0	Sports	Racquetball, general
10.0	Running	Running, 6mph	10.0	Sports	Rope jumping, general
11.0	Running	Running, 6.7mph	10.0	Sports	Rugby
11.5	Running	Running, 7mph	5.0	Sports	Skateboarding
12.5	Running	Running, 7.5mph	7.0	Sports	Skating, roller
13.5	Running	Running, 8mph	3.5	Sports	Sky diving
14.0	Running	Running, 8.6mph	7.0	Sports	Soccer, general
15.0	Running	Running, 9mph	5.0	Sports	Baseball, general
16.0	Running	Running, 10mph	12.0	Sports	Squash
18.0	Running	Running, 10.9mph	4.0	Sports	Table tennis
9.0	Running	Running, cross country	4.0	Sports	Tai chi
8.0	Running	Running, general	7.0	Sports	Tennis, general
8.0	Running	Running, in place	3.0	Sports	Volleyball, general
15.0	Running	Running, stairs, up	6.0	Sports	Wrestling (5min)
10.0	Running	Running, on a track	2.0	Transportation	Automobile, driving, light
3.0	Running	Running, wheeling, general	2.5	Transportation	Motor cycle
2.5	Self-Care	Standing-preparing for bed	3.0	Transportation	Driving heavy truck
1.0	Self-Care	Sitting on toilet	7.0	Walking	Backpacking, general

METS	CATEGORY	SPECIFIC ACTIVITY
9.0	Walking	Carrying load upstairs, general
3.0	Walking	Downstairs
6.0	Walking	Hiking, cross country
6.5	Walking	Marching, rapidly, military
6.5	Walking	Race walking
8.0	Walking	Rock/mountain climbing
8.0	Walking	Up stairs, climbing up ladder
4.0	Walking	Using crutches
2.0	Walking	Walking, <2.0mph
3.0	Walking	Walking, 2.5mph, firm surface
3.0	Walking	Walking, 2.5mph, downhill
3.5	Walking	Walking, 3.0mph, moderate
4.0	Walking	Walking, 3.5mph
6.0	Walking	Walking, 3.5mph, uphill
4.0	Walking	Walking, 4.0mph, very brisk
4.5	Walking	Walking, 4.5mph, very brisk
3.5	Walking	Walking, for pleasure
5.0	Walking	Walking, to work or class
3.5	Water Activities	Canoeing, rowing, general
3.0	Water Activities	Diving, springboard
5.0	Water Activities	Kayaking
4.0	Water Activities	Paddleboat
3.0	Water Activities	Sailing, general
7.0	Water Activities	Skin diving, general
5.0	Water Activities	Snorkeling
3.0	Water Activities	Surfing
10.0	Water Activities	Swimming, breaststroke general
11.0	Water Activities	Swimming, butterfly, general
6.0	Water Activities	Swimming, leisurely, general
10.0	Water Activities	Water polo
3.0	Water Activities	Water volleyball
7.0	Winter Activities	Skating, ice, general
7.0	Winter Activities	Skiing, general
5.0	Winter Activities	Skiing, downhill, light
6.0	Winter Activities	Skiing, downhill, moderate
8.0	Winter Activities	Skiing, downhill, vigorous
7.0	Winter Activities	Sledding, tobogganing, bobsled
8.0	Winter Activities	Snow shoeing
3.5	Winter Activities	Snowmobiling